Competition and Planning in the NHS

Competition and Planning in the NHS

THE CONSEQUENCES OF THE NHS REFORMS

SECOND EDITION

Calum Paton

Professor of Health Policy
Keele University

with

Kevin Hunt
Katherine Birch **Kelvin Jordan**

Stanley Thornes (Publishers) Ltd

First edition published by Chapman & Hall in 1992
(ISBN 0-412-47060-8)

Second edition published in 1998 by:
Stanley Thornes (Publishers) Ltd
Ellenborough House
Wellington Street
CHELTENHAM
GL50 1YW
United Kingdom

98 99 00 01 / 10 9 8 7 6 5 4 3 2 1

A catalogue record for this book is available from the British Library

ISBN 0-7487-3307-8

Typeset by Acorn Bookwork, Salisbury, Wiltshire
Printed and bound in Great Britain by
T.J. International Ltd, Padstow, Cornwall

FOR MY DAUGHTER, LEAH

Contents

Preface vii

Acknowledgements ix

Introduction 1

1 **The consequences of the reforms: where we are today** 6

2 **Ideology, right-wing ideas and conservative reforms: the Prime Minister's Review** 18

3 **Central features of the NHS reforms** 39
(Contributor: Lynn Ashburner)

4 **The market, the purchaser/provider split, and contracting: surveys and case studies** 66
(Co-authors: Kevin Hunt, Kelvin Jordan and Katherine Birch)

5 **Purchasing: new vintage or just new label?** 109
(Contributors: Katherine Birch, Joan Durose and Debbie Harrison)

6 **The consequences revisited** 132

7 **The future** 162

References 181

Key agencies 186

Index 187

Preface

This is the second edition of a book published in 1992, entitled *Competition and Planning in the NHS*, with a subtitle then of *The Danger of Unplanned Markets*. The aim was to explain the antecedents to the NHS reforms and the reforms themselves, in terms of both British politics and debates within health care. The book went on to set out the likely consequences of the reforms at the general level, based on close analysis of the content of the reforms at that stage. The general prediction was that the reforms posed clear dangers for an NHS geared to meeting need equitably and economically.

This second edition is almost wholly rewritten, with only one chapter (Chapter 2) retained from the first edition (and that updated where necessary). This is inevitable as well as desirable. For the reforms have evolved, up to 1997, into a complex web of initiatives which both require new analysis and also cry out for overall evaluation.

This book works in the spirit of the original edition, not least in taking as the central question whether competition and 'the market' had infused the NHS by 1997. Alternatively, did 'planning' and central control remain salient albeit disguised in new language and using new mechanisms and structures?

This edition moves on, however, to evaluate crucial aspects of the reforms and to trace their likely consequences for the health service of the future. In doing the latter, it explores *inter alia* how the Labour Party's health policy evolved to cope with the *fait accompli* of the reforms, as well as how the Conservative Party's agenda shaped the new NHS. In the light of Labour's 1997 election victory, the reconciliation of needs-based planning with the policies and structures inherited by Labour has become problematical and the final pages of this book point to some of the tensions.

The evaluation is the first to draw on both detailed empirical research and policy analysis from a vantage point of more than five years after the initial implementation of the reforms. The aim of the evaluative part is overtly to judge 'the whole' as well as some of the key 'parts'. The prognosis for the future, while based on personal judgement as well, is thus grounded in research and informed commentary at a number of levels.

The empirical research was generously funded by the Nuffield Trust, under a major grant of which the author was the grantholder and director of the resulting project.

Taken together, editions one and two tell the story of the NHS reforms, up to the time when a new government in 1997 altered the emphasis (if not radically). While the reader must be the judge, many of the predictions made in 1992 arguably came about, although the exact policies and structures and particular debates 'live' then have changed considerably. Hence, again, the need for a wholly new book, albeit geared to addressing the same tension created by the NHS reforms – that between competitive markets and social planning.

Chapter 1 sets out where we are today – some (often unintended or, rather, unanticipated) consequences of the reforms, which will take some years to alter even if such an attempt is made. That is, the film starts with a glimpse of the dénouement. This is the reality against which to judge the intentions and pretensions analysed in Chapters 2 and 3. Chapters 4 and 5 present specific evaluations of central aspects of the reforms and therefore (Chapter 4 especially) report empirical results. Their style is therefore more 'researchy' than the narrative of all the other chapters – including Chapters 6 and 7, which explore the implications for the future.

Acknowledgements

One chapter is co-authored. Two others carry contributions from the team assembled to carry out the empirical research. This was funded by the Nuffield Trust in a grant to Professor Paton, who is Professor of Health Policy, Centre for Health Planning and Management, Keele University. All the co-authors are faculty members of the Centre for Health Planning and Management, Keele University, along with Professor Paton. Katherine Birch is Research Assistant and a medical sociologist. Kevin Hunt is Research Fellow and a health economist. Kelvin Jordan is Research Fellow and a statistician.

Dr Lynn Ashburner is Lecturer in Management, Keele University, and author of books and articles on NHS organisation and boards. Joan Durose, Executive Director, Combined Healthcare, Staffordshire (a community trust) and PhD student at the Centre for Health Planning and Management, Keele, and Debbie Harrison MBA (Health Executive), Centre for Health Planning and Management, Keele, contributed some research materials for Chapter 5. Additionally, Clare Jinks, Research Fellow, Keele, and Lynn Ashburner – along with the co-authors – undertook some of the case studies, lessons from which are summarised at the end of Chapter 4.

Finally, I would like to thank Barbara Goodenough, Office Manager at the Centre, for organising the production of this manuscript, including much typing. I would also like to thank my partner Tracey and baby daughter Leah for feigning an occasional interest in the continuing saga of the NHS reforms.

Introduction

While there are many technical evaluations of particular aspects of the NHS reforms, independent evaluation of broader consequences has been missing. An earlier study by the King's Fund (Robinson and Le Grand, 1994) reviewed particular initiatives and institutions associated with the reforms, but at an earlier stage when the emerging contours of the overall consequences were less visible. Naturally no study can evaluate everything, but the rationale for this book is broad-based evaluation. It also presents analysis of some specific aspects of the reforms: in particular, the purchaser/provider split, the market and contracting (Chapter 4) and the question of whether new priorities have emerged through 'purchasing' in the National Health Service (Chapter 5). It also provides informed assessment and commentary on the most salient trends in British health care which are associated with the reforms.

This leads to another point. It would be irresponsible, if not impossible, to attribute specific outcomes to specific causes in a pseudo-scientific manner, when so many changes have occurred together. It has already been pointed out on a number of occasions that the implementation of the reforms, prior to the 1992 general election, was accompanied by infusion of money to 'grease the wheels' of the reform process. Thus, when it comes to (for example) considering increased productivity or greater workload in the service, it is well-nigh impossible to disentangle the effects of changed incentives and institutions following the reforms, on the one hand, and 'good old-fashioned extra cash', on the other hand.

Additionally, the NHS reforms have become all things to all men. Many evolutionary trends already existing within the service became associated with the reforms after the White Paper, *Working for Patients*, was published in 1989 and after the implementation of the 1990 NHS Act on 1st April 1991.

Even the new policy initiatives which were directly part of *Working for Patients* are too numerous to allow exact attribution of cause and effect. On the one hand there is 'the market', or the alleged market; there is the purchaser/provider split (a phrase not used in the White Paper) as distinct from the market; there are the specifics of the contracting process; there are institutions such as NHS trusts and new types of purchasing agency, including GP fundholding. Beyond this, there are other policy initiatives which do not stem directly from *Working for Patients* but are now considered to be part of the NHS reforms. Among the latter can be numbered Patient's Charter initiatives; the *Health of the Nation* policy; and the more recent aspiration to move to a 'primary care-led NHS', whatever that means in practice.

All of these initiatives have gradually become immersed into a series of instructions to health authorities (and other purchasers) from government, sometimes acting through regional health authorities – regional offices after 1st April 1996. Indeed, a basic point in policy analysis arises here. It is difficult both conceptually and practically to distinguish between policy and implementation. The policy document heralding the NHS reforms, *Working for Patients*, was – unlike some previous blueprints for structural reform of the NHS, as in 1974 and 1982 – a thin document. It was easily digestible at the theoretical level yet required much 'policy making on the hoof' from 1989 (and particularly 1991) onwards. To this extent it had a precedent in the Griffiths Report of October 1983, which was also a thin document with significant consequences for the managerial reorganisation of the service. The reforms, however, went significantly further.

In other words, in order to implement such policy, it is necessary to continue the process of making policy. The question therefore arises, who does it? Even the use of the word 'reform' is not value neutral. Reform often has positive prescriptive overtones: the implication is that the old system was bad and needed reform.

This raises another highly related point: there is a specific political agenda behind the NHS reforms. All policy is political (in France and many other countries, the same word is used for 'politics' and 'policy' – *la politique*). In Britain, although we tend to have a stiffer upper lip in distinguishing politics and administration (if not implementation), the point remains, nonetheless.

The NHS reforms can be described, without exaggeration, as having a political core and also a technical core. The two must be distinguished, although often with difficulty. The political core to the NHS reforms was an ideological belief in market mechanisms and an opposition to state planning and traditional patterns of state financing and provision (in health care as elsewhere in the economy). The technical element of the reforms concerns mechanisms for achieving objectives – for example, contracting systems and aspects of the purchaser/provider split which are seen (perhaps naively) as politically neutral. Debates within the latter realm often spill over into debates within the former realm, as for example government ministers often seek to justify the former agenda by reference to the latter, hiding political decisions within seemingly technical matters.

The timescale for evaluating the consequences of the NHS reforms is, of course, important. NHS managers were asked to do it after a year; political scientists assume we should wait about 20 years; and one is reminded of Chairman Mao's reply, when asked for his assessment of the French Revolution, that it was too early to tell! To a certain extent it is 'horses for courses'. Smaller scale, well-defined innovations can be evaluated in a more self-contained manner, whereas longer term consequences for the health service as a whole of particular policies and of their political consequences are arguably more important. This book is completed almost nine years after the Prime Minister's Review of the National Health Service which led to the transformations known as the NHS reforms, and certain consequences are now becoming apparent. Some of these are planned. Some are unplanned and unanticipated, as contradictory policies are reconciled in an *ad hoc* manner according to political agendas as well as to the need to iron out incompatible trends.

While we must be careful about comparative health policy analysis, considering trends in other countries can help to give us a picture of our own wood as well as the trees within it. One paradox, which arises when considering the origin of the NHS reforms, concerns whether they were unique or common to a whole range of European and other countries. The paradox is that both seem true. The British reform process was instituted by Lady Thatcher at the beginning of 1988 when interviewed on *Panorama*. She sought to make attack the best form of defence when being asked about apparent funding problems in the National Health Service over the winter of 1987–88. Thus was the Review of the National Health Service announced. That gives it a uniquely British flavour.

On the other hand, there are few health care systems which are not undergoing reform, and the phrase 'health sector reform' is now much in vogue not just in Europe, North America and beyond, but throughout the 'underdeveloped' world as well. To some extent this is fad and fashion – new languages quickly move from one country to another, often carried directly in the briefing documents and consultancy papers which international advisers take around the world (Marmor, 1997).

There is, however, another explanation – the mismatch between expectations of health services and available resources is growing sharper, for a number of reasons. These include the familiar litany of changing demography; advancing technology; medical sector inflation; new pandemics such as AIDS; and the decline of the extended, self-protecting family in Western society.

At the level of political economy, however, another major explanation exists: the global capitalist economy has developed in such a manner that low tax and low public expenditure are the orthodoxy of the age. Capital has to be attracted and individual countries are part of an international auction for investment and jobs. In this environment, pressure on government expenditure, and public health services in particular, is great. This transcends traditional party politics organised within the nation state, although of course Conservative governments have hitherto been more in tune with this evolving trend.

As a result, there is an overwhelming pressure upon public health services, and therefore a sense that 'the old ways' are inadequate to cope. To this extent, any reform process is about productivity and what our transatlantic cousins would call 'getting more bang for the buck'.

There is one major, superficially surprising, point of consensus in interpreting the intentions behind the British reform. Its supporters argue that the aim was to change the terms of debate from 'more money for the NHS' to 'what we do with the available money'. Lady Thatcher used the graphic phrase 'black hole' about the old NHS's financing system; money was poured in, she alleged, without being properly accounted for in terms of output. Thus, instead of more money, the reform process would focus upon targeting existing money. Opponents of the reforms would agree with this diagnosis. They would cast it in a different prescriptive light, however, and often argue that the agenda was about cutting public expenditure and favouring gradual privatisation of health provision – and to some extent health financing as well.

The succeeding analysis will paint some of the institutions created by the NHS reforms as having a political function as well as a more neutral managerial or economic function. That is, the aim was to prevent major interests and institutions within the NHS from having what former Minister of Health Enoch Powell had called at the beginning of the 1960s a vested interest in denigration of the service – that is, pleas for more money to solve alleged problems and meet alleged shortfalls. Instead, a dynamic is created whereby purchasers haggle with providers over static budgets. This has the useful functions of 'divide and rule' and devolving responsibility for the money. That was both the intention and the operation of the new system. And the 'internal market' was bound to be costly to operate. Even when health authorities and provider trusts were forced by regional offices to restrict local market transactions (see Chapter 1), the costs of GP fundholding, short-term contracting and individual patient billing for 'extra contractual referrals' (see later chapters) were high. The latter aspects are what the Labour Party seemed to refer to in its 1997 campaign as 'the internal market'. For by 1997 there was no recognisable competitive market involving major trusts competing for large-scale health authority contracts. Regional planning took precedence.

So, in the end, the new NHS is not a market (either real or mimic) but a new type of political planning, with more top-down control than ever before. If we must invoke dramatic analogies, it is Stalin rather than Adam Smith – the visible fist, not the invisible hand! The defeat of the Conservatives in 1997 does not, however, alter the fact that the mechanics of the NHS reforms are well entrenched (deliberately so) and would take time to 'unpick', even were this attempted. Omelettes are not easily unscrambled.

1 The consequences of the reforms: where we are today

INTRODUCTION

To some, the NHS reforms mean everything that has happened in the health service since 1990. To others, they mean the introduction of a market system into the provision of health care. This study steers a middle course between these two definitions, focusing on a number of key changes to be discussed in the following paragraphs.

Given the nature and content of the reforms, no simple evaluation – and certainly not a quantitative one – is possible. This is not a 'cop-out': indeed, the aim is to delineate more usefully what a study such as the present one can offer, in terms of both assessing the reforms and making recommendations for the future of the NHS. Evaluation implies judgement as well as data. While judgement is bound to contain elements of subjectivity, informed judgement ought to be able to provide perspective or relation of trends to consequences and likely implications for the future of public health care in Britain.

As suggested above, when asked what one thinks of the NHS reforms, one is reminded of Chairman Mao's alleged dictum, when asked what he thought of the French Revolution, that it was 'too early to tell'. For managers acting at the behest of the government of the day, the reforms could be evaluated (for partisan purposes) a year or two after being implemented. Managers could justify this rather meaningless assessment by defining success in terms of implementing new processes and structures. At the other extreme, for the political scientist, a period of 20–25 years is perhaps nearer the mark in terms of evaluating the consequences of the reforms for the direction of services and policy. Yet again, this study seeks the middle way: which new trends can be identified as a result of the reforms? Whether the importance of new trends is increased or diminished over time is, of course, a matter for the longer term.

To make this point sharply: were the reforms merely the most recent in an increasingly long line of administrative reorganisations within the National Health Service or are they the enabling catalyst for the abandonment of consensus around the provision of a universal, comprehensive and egalitarian public health service?

This is not simply a revisiting of the pre-1992 question, 'Is the internal market in the NHS about privatisation?'. In an immediate technical sense, the answer has been initially 'No', with the fairly major exception of the Private Finance Initiative (PFI), which is facilitated by the existence of self-governing hospitals and other providers which are not part of an integrated health authority. In a broader sense, however, the NHS reforms are but one small part of the political evolution from the late 1980s, revisiting the foundations of public finance and in particular the welfare state (including the health service). Viewed from this perspective, the reforms may be both consequence and cause – a response to the pressures within and on public health services and a series of mechanisms which have a knock-on effect as regards new health policies and, indeed, new ways of making health policy. In evaluating the reforms, it is therefore important to seek to assess (however imperfectly) such dynamic factors as well as more static issues (such as the productivity of hospitals following new contracting systems and the like).

In outlining key consequences of the reforms in the opening chapter, this book runs the risk of the kind of artistic licence claimed by films which begin with the ending. Since the reforms are not, however, a closed book, nor a simple episode in which a clear conclusion follows from a limited number of measurable beginnings, it is perhaps as well to set out the overall observations, against which can be set more detailed findings reported later in the book. Additionally, given that the origins and content of the reforms have now been fully debated, it is interesting to set evolving consequences against initial assumptions. That is, what has been intended; what has been unintended, by whom?

FINANCING THE NHS – THE POLITICAL ECONOMY OF HEALTH CARE

The NHS reforms were implemented without changing the mechanism for financing the NHS overall; in other words, mainly through general taxation. Nevertheless, the tax system had become markedly less progressive through the 1980s. In consequence, the tax burden underlying public expenditure had shifted. More after-tax income was in the hands of the better off than previously and this had implications for financing health care as well as other services. For example, more disposable income in the hands of the better off led to an incremental but significant growth in private health insurance and purchase of private health care. Simply to finance the NHS (and other government expenditure programmes) at the same level meant a relatively greater tax burden on the less well off, with the consequence that it became politically more difficult to increase taxes without hitting the less well off taxpayers.

A political consensus around fewer taxes (certainly direct taxes) may be interpreted as what Galbraith has called 'the politics of the contented majority' (Galbraith, 1992). Right-of-centre electoral majorities are now more easily composed of 'the better-off two-thirds'. The tax burden is (relatively) shifted to the poor, if not reduced overall, and as a result neither richer nor poorer is willing to see tax rises to finance increased government expenditure. To put it no doubt simplistically, the politics of the 1960s and early 1970s had seen competition between the political parties to increase government expenditure. The politics of the 1980s and 1990s were, however, to be about competition to cut taxes. The new political orthodoxy was shaped by widespread belief that in the international economy, only a policy of low taxation was compatible with the kind of enterprise economy required to attract inward investment. Capital was international and mobile, aided by new information technology amongst other things: national labour forces were in competition with each other, as the balance of power between capital and labour shifted in favour of the former.

In consequence, perceptions that public expenditure had to be limited were sharpened and bolstered. Pressure on funding of the welfare state led, in the case of health care, to a belief that allegedly voracious, if not infinite, demand for services would have to be financed by dramatically increased productivity. In other words, the debate should turn from pleas for more money to examination of the efficiency and effectiveness of existing expenditure.

On this point, both proponents and opponents of the NHS reforms were agreed: when Mrs Thatcher announced a 'fundamental review' of the National Health Service, it was intended to change the terms of debate in exactly such a direction (Paton, 1992).

Public health services are frequently viewed in two ways. On the one hand, they are means of providing universal services in as egalitarian a manner as possible. On the other hand, they are economical means of investing in a healthy workforce. It would be too simplistic to describe these different perspectives as the 'consumption' and 'investment' views respectively, but the latter view was behind a developing orientation towards judging health-care programmes in terms not only of clinical outcome but also of economic and social outcome. And if efficiency were to be judged in terms of labour productivity (with labour costs 70% of the NHS's total costs), then seeking to meet demand through increased productivity would mean either greater efficiency from or greater exploitation of professionals and workers in the NHS.

THE SPIRIT OF THE REFORMS

None of this proves that the NHS reforms were rationally designed to meet such long-term objectives. But it does suggest that, in shaping the reforms over time, this could become the longer term agenda. That is, in common with other countries, pressures on expenditure would grow.

Mechanisms for dealing with this pressure would of course vary, not least because political systems and domestic political pressures infusing health services would vary. It has already been said, for example, that the internal market was an answer awaiting a question, a solution awaiting a problem (Paton, 1992). The institutions and mechanisms created by such political initiatives were always likely, however, to be co-opted in the longer term, to a more clearly perceived agenda. *Ad hoc* reactions may throw up possibilities; 'cock-ups' can be used in emerging conspiracies.

It was not the theology of the market, internal or otherwise, which was to be important in the long term. Both our surveys and our case studies undertaken systematically over four years suggest that belief in the market was both limited and transient, at the highest level, although ironically managers in the National Health Service came to believe the rhetoric preached by their political masters. More important was the need to shape the institutions of the reformed NHS 'to do more with less' – paradoxically, even when these institutions *per se* were often created at great expense.

When competition between hospital trusts was useful in reducing the wage bill, for example, it might well be encouraged. Equally, if it became expensive and disruptive of other priorities, good old-fashioned planning was often readmitted, but through the back door. If competition cut costs, it was to be encouraged. When it did the opposite, things were rather different. Nor was it simply a question of labour costs. The contracting systems which developed with the implementation of the reforms meant that the new purchasers often sought deals 'at the margin'. In aggregate, this often meant that total costs, and capital costs, were underfunded, but in the short term this seemed like 'efficiency'. Coupled with pricing rules which developed as part of the regulation of the market, efficiency became defined as low unit costs and the more efficient a provider unit (hospital or community service) became, the more it was expected to do within a static budgetary total. This was not so much a free market as a year-on-year squeeze on resources, by central regulation.

A number of factors, both immediate and longer term, came to influence the path taken by the reforms. The fiscal politics underlying NHS expenditure changed somewhat. As a result, greater squeeze upon both labour and capital resources was sought. Aspects of the new market, and in particular new contracting systems, were used in pursuit of such squeeze. And yet the formal content of the reforms – self-governing trusts, a purchaser/provider split, GP fundholding and the like – could by no means be seen as part of a rational plan to provide a leaner NHS. Instead, initiative upon initiative followed the initial implementation of the reforms in 1991. Taken literally or even imaginatively, many of these initiatives contradicted each other. The manner in which they were reconciled (of necessity) represented the sense in which immediate, opportunistic political initiatives could be shaped to meet longer term ends. To put it another way, if one were asked whether the reforms represented a series of policy fragments or a rational plan – alternatively, 'cock-up' or 'conspiracy' – the answer would have to be both. Particular initiatives were not part of a master plan – anything but. Yet, longer term agendas shaped the manner in which particular initiatives were hammered together. Problems from contradictory policies were 'thrown up' in the implementation process. Yet most of the decision making to reconcile these was central.

An illustration helps. The central plank of the reforms provided a market in health care, based on a split between the purchaser (both health authority and, within it, GP fundholders) and provider (hospital and community units) and upon systems for making contracts between purchasers and providers. Without going fully into the necessary and sufficient conditions for markets to be effective, it was clear that certain characteristics would have to obtain if the new market were to live up to its pretensions. Providers would have to be free to make their own decisions as to when, how and to what extent to seek new investment. Purchasers would make their own decisions as to where to place contracts for services, with patients then being referred in line with these contracts. This is just a common-sense way of stating the economist's prescription that provider markets must be adequately competitive and that there should not be an imbalance of power between the purchaser and provider. (For example, a monopolistic provider or monopsonistic (single) purchaser would prevent the advantages of markets obtaining.)

In practice, however, the institutions and mechanisms for contracting, and the contracting process itself, are a major source of both 'planning blight' and additional management costs in the NHS. Marketing by separate providers; duplication of function and staff by provider and purchaser; local purchasers with different agendas, based on faulty assumptions about their neighbouring purchasers' intentions; the proliferation of GP fundholders; contract preparation on both sides; monitoring, disputing, billing and then recontracting annually: all these are productive of both a fragmented health service and high costs, as our case studies and questionnaires respectively suggest.

Additionally, devolving such contracting to GPs, whether full fundholders or not (but especially if the former), increases cost considerably. In one of our case studies, GP fundholders provided 10% of the budget to a clinical directorate but incurred 90% of the management costs. And these are just direct management costs. From one surgical directorate (in a large hospital in the West Midlands), fundholders sought and obtained outpatient clinics at their surgeries rather than the hospital. This sounded nice and no doubt was, for a minority of patients. Yet the clinical director estimated that for ten patients seen this way, he could have seen 70 at the hospital.

At the strategic level, the natural catchment areas for many types of hospital treatment are greater than health authorities, so leaving purchasing and contracting to health authorities (even the new, larger ones) may lead to incompatible decisions. Authority A may decide to move contracts, for example, to Hospital X from Y, on the basis that Authority B already finances X and that therefore economies of scale (and lower prices) may be forthcoming. But if Authority B is meanwhile (in blissful ignorance) transferring contracts to Hospital Y on the basis that A funds it already (on the same logic!) then neither will achieve their objectives. Both authorities and hospitals will simply switch their business. No economies of scale will be forthcoming.

And, if rationalisation such as merger would produce a benefit, who is to organise it if it requires super-authority action? The reforms have over-devolved purchasing or, rather, necessitated back-door planning as a prerequisite step to purchasing. This is not revealed by 'surveys' but is a central consequence of the reforms.

As a result, policy makers were required to intervene not so much merely to 'manage the market' as to plan the service, but behind the closed doors of regional 'market meetings' (a term used in the West Midlands). Purchasers' intentions had to be co-ordinated; providers' likewise; then purchasers with providers; heads knocked together if necessary. Planning – a rose by any other name (but more expensive)?

As this process emerged, ministers and senior managers began to see that a combination of central planning and local 'market pressure' could force costs down; at street level, providers would vie viciously, but in an auction to survive by best pleasing the planners. A nice British compromise or divide and rule?

Such cost can only be justified by reference to greater benefit such as increased effectiveness of the service or greater efficiency, to outweigh the cost. But if the NHS is a service which seeks to meet need in an egalitarian manner, it cannot operate in such a way.

ASSESSMENT OF THE REFORMS – COMPETITION OR PLANNING?

Direct measurement of both total cost and 'benefit' before and after the reforms is impossible, as organisational structures (including the development of clinical directorates) have changed so much in parallel with the reforms. Additionally, data on 'output' from hospital departments are not available in commensurate form, pre- and post-reform. Finally, even were it possible, to compare cost and changes in output does not allow an easy attribution of cause and effect (Le Grand, 1994).

Nevertheless, the additional 'management' costs of the new NHS are not easily justified in terms of their contribution to new services or more justifiable priorities. These costs are largely administrative; they are not managerial in the strategic sense. The new NHS is marked by more centralism than ever, especially in directing health authorities and trusts as to priorities and meeting targets set by indicators, including the Patient's Charter.

As a result, achieving objectives set from above, through mechanisms originally justified as necessary to run a decentralised market from below, is a cumbersome administrative task. Instead of being an integrated, streamlined organisation, the NHS in its local incarnation has to work through contract and negotiation yet without the corresponding freedom in terms of which the market was justified.

When a regional office (acting on behalf of the government) wants to rationalise accident and emergency services, it has to 'knock purchasers' heads together'. Purchasers, in turn, have to deal indirectly with providers. 'Self-governing' trusts see their role as preserving autonomy, yet this may fly in the face of service requirements, in particular rationalisation (BBC *Panorama*, January 6, 1997).

'New priorities' by local purchasers are revealed by our surveys as relatively insignificant, unless new central government 'initiatives' are defined as new priorities locally. The costs of the new purchasing function *per se,* as well as of the purchaser/provider split (Paton, 1996; Ch 7, pp133–6), are difficult to justify in terms of innovation or more appropriate expenditure.

What is more, increased 'efficiency', in the sense of productivity, is largely achieved (where it is at all) through use of the market to discipline the professions and labour force. Lower wages and intensified labour are not increased organisational efficiency. There may be more output for the same cost (or less, with annual 'efficiency savings' of 3%) but this is achieved through central directives on pricing policy and through local contracting which does not cover full costs. 'Local pay' provides another example. Local pay is in truth centrally set pay, with centrally set rules concerning local additions (if any) to national decisions. Any 'efficiency' gained by holding pay below inflation is the result of central decision making.

The most significant evolving consequence of the reforms, detectable by 1996–97, is the use of an expanded and more expensive management cadre to put downward pressure on the costs of 'front-line' care. (This is the media's 'grey suits instead of doctors and nurses'.) And later, when new policies and pressures have been set in train, it is then possible to reduce the management cadre itself. Hence the Secretary of State's directives to reduce management costs in 1995 and 1996, ironically despite their origin as the price of running the market. The Labour Party has followed this line – put pressure on management costs, but retain the institutions of the purchaser/provider split which cause many of the costs! The election victory of 1997 is likely to lead to a central 'task force' to seek savings. But these will be difficult without yet more radical reorganisation, which Labour wishes to avoid.

Both proponents and opponents of the reforms, again, can agree that this is the evolving intention, even if the 'whats and hows' were not planned in 1991. Increasing pressure is the name of the game, whether one approves or disapproves. The further development of a low tax economy depends on it.

Planning of services is dominated by providers and by regional offices or the central NHS Executive itself. Health authorities are squeezed in the middle. This is ironic because 'strong purchasing' was allegedly a major intention of the reforms. It had itself, however, been a post-hoc rationalisation after 1992, when the district health authority was to be the jewel in the crown of the reforms. And, in time, this flavour of the year went stale: by the end of 1994, 'strong purchasing' was allegedly devolved to GPs, as set out in the NHS Executive document of October 1994, *Towards a Primary-Care Led NHS*. In reality, GPs' roles were not to plan services but to haggle over deals once services had been planned and provided. The key planning decisions were taken regionally and centrally. So the search for the *deus ex machina* of the reforms continued.

The 'primary health care-led NHS' seemed ready-made for the role. It is a means of offering greater 'consumer choice' as regards relatively minor frills, while putting further financial pressure on hospitals by transferring certain secondary services into the community (either directly provided or locally purchased by GP fundholders, or GP commissioning groups after 1998). It is also based on the assumption that more spending on 'primary care' will reduce pressure on secondary care, a highly dubious assumption. Only a utopian strategy to prevent ill health could achieve this. Even then, primary care supply might create its own secondary care demand.

The NHS reforms have therefore become a series of centrally promulgated changes. A 'policy for everything', and seemingly a new initiative a month, became the norm. Part of the political motivation was, of course, to wrong-foot the opposition, by creating an omelette which cannot be unscrambled.

As a result, by 1997, the Labour Party had moved to a position of accepting nearly all the institutions of the new NHS yet promising savings by 'abolishing the market'. To make significant savings would, however, require a simplified structure and streamlined planning process. This in turn would involve removing the rigidities of the purchaser/provider split, replacing the myriad 'purchasing' arrangements and contracts with a regional planning process which linked resources to agreed levels of service for populations and only sparingly involving GP representatives in this planning process, as well as other experts.

Instead, seeking to be 'realistic' and 'forward-looking' and fearing accusations of 'turning back the clock', Labour might actually increase the complexity of the present system. This could occur if it seeks to decentralise 'commissioning' to all GPs (admittedly, it proposed to replace 3000 GP fundholding groups with 500 local commissioning groups) and to build further rigidity into the purchaser/provider split (unintentionally) by 'democratising' trust boards and therefore making local services less easily malleable by planners. In this context, 'abolishing the market' would not mean significant cost saving, except for that achieved by longer term contracts and less fundholding costs.

CONTRACTS AND MARKET INCENTIVES – LOCAL DECISIONS OR DIKTAT?

Our surveys reveal that most contracts between purchaser and provider are still block contracts, although with a trend to more sophisticated versions with 'floors and ceilings'. Additionally, an overwhelming conclusion is that most referrals are still to local providers except where the planning process has closed these. The internal market has not resulted in radically new criteria for referral or patient choice to travel further.

As a result, the main use of contracting has been as a financial stick for purchasers. A 'textbook' market would allow providers to seek alternative purchasers, as well as purchasers seeking alternative providers. In practice, however, financially squeezed providers require each fragment of income they can get. (By 1996, many acute trusts were 'in the red' or forced to limit non-urgent admissions early in the financial year.) As a result, a multiplicity of purchasers does not increase provider power, except in rare cases.

Purchasers tend to have money but not detailed information as to clinical services. They have therefore used their bargaining power not to challenge priorities between or within clinical departments, but to cut costs. Purchasers now have power without responsibility (for implementing the consequences of their decisions, as when health authorities had responsibility for providers).

A significant additional consequence of having both a purchaser/provider split and separate, local providers facing more direct financial pressures and incentives is that providers often seek to 'pass the buck' to each other. Local 'seamless' care is adversely affected when hospitals have to seek early discharge to meet contractual and financial requirements. Co-ordination of care between hospital and community becomes a matter for contractual intricacy to link separate organisations, mandated by purchasers often without adequate information. Analogies exist with other (formerly) public sector organisations, such as the railways, where separate, commercial companies, previously within an integrated network, make journeys more complex and fragmented. It makes sense to have an amicable separation between hospital and community services, as long as they continue to live in the same house. Separate management units were more clearly created following the Griffiths Inquiry of 1983. But, following the reforms, this separation has become a divorce. An agency to co-ordinate separate providers seems to be lacking and, ironically, this was the role played by the district health authority prior to 1991. Otherwise, purchasers and providers are forced by financial incentives and by the pressure from myriad government directives to squeeze more from the system; to pass the buck to each other (Paton, 1995). Labour's policy, post-1997, of rationalising provision lacks a stable mechanism to achieve it.

Another consequence of separate, quasi-commercial providers was that each must break even, and make a 6% return on capital, in each financial year. As with purchasing, this may well involve overdecentralisation: expecting trusts to break even over a longer period of time, and on a larger scale, may make more commercial sense, let alone more sense for a public service. Few businesses are expected to make a standard rate of return, in every division, every year. A sensible planning process for the NHS would take a longer and wider view.

What is more, the public capital programme for the NHS has virtually disappeared. Most capital is now expected to be private. Yet the payback of this capital has to come from the public, NHS budget. Forcing a 'return' on capital is not in practice the smack of market discipline but a means of forcing providers to cut costs further, so they can charge purchasers less and so that in turn the NHS (purchasers') budget can then seemingly cope. In practice, seeking a surplus (return on capital) is a means of diktat whereby services are assumed to be funded to cover their capital costs and pay capital charges, even when they are not. In other words, says government, 'We're no longer funding capital, but you hospitals must budget for it'.

Fragmentation into many purchasers has created consequences for both providers and public which contravene hitherto accepted norms for the NHS. Firstly, inequity may be systematised. Although the 'old NHS' saw variations in access according to geography, location and local organisation, the aim was explicitly to reduce this. Now, access depends on the finance available to a smaller purchaser and whether or not that purchaser is more generously funded (*ceteris paribus*) than others. Secondly, financial squeeze is not only increasing on providers but affects the public differentially. Referrals now have to follow contracts and the 'financial nexus' is more direct. 'Stop–go' occurs, whereby sanctioned referrals and treatment dry up and restart suddenly, according to whether or not the purchaser has run out of money. This seems arbitrary to the public. What is more, it is no use for providers: they may have reached financial crisis, before stop suddenly becomes go again. Valuable services can be lost between the cracks.

Extracontractual referrals (ECRs) became expensive to administer and were a very bureaucratic means of handling what (in the 'old NHS') were straightforward free referrals. Both the former government (following a review by the NHS Efficiency Unit reporting in March 1996) and the new Labour government were pledged to 'end' ECRs, but at the cost of **more** bureaucracy, i.e. by regulating and seeking to 'second guess' referrals or by simply planning contracts in line with observed referrals. To do the latter is simply to replicate the 'old NHS' but more bureaucratically – an irony, given that proponents of the internal market had set up the Aunt Sally of bureaucratic hierarchies, and 'command and control', in the old NHS.

In aggregate, these trends within and consequences of the reforms give power to accusations that spending on bureaucracy has increased at the cost of patient care. Some decisions may be more overt and more linking of outcome and cost may indeed be sought. But it is at least questionable whether the latter consequences outweigh the cost and, indeed, whether the latter consequences are more benign than the 'informality' of the old NHS. Overt purchasing is not necessarily more rational purchasing or planning. Linking outcome and cost is only as good as the methodology and the values governing its uses. And the market has no logical link with health authorities' policies to link outcome and cost. It is perfectly possible to plan directly managed services on that basis and then allow referral to them.

In consequence, recouping expanded management costs is often at the cost of greater pressure on front-line services.

COMPETITION, MANAGED COMPETITION, CONTESTABILITY OR NONE OF THESE?

The mainstream debate about the market, following the NHS reforms, concerned whether or not it was a real competitive market (albeit in the public sector), a 'managed market' or merely a potential market (with providers only replaced in extreme circumstances, as a result of their position being stable yet 'contestable' in the last instance).

The conclusions reported in this book, however, suggest it was none of these. Clearly it is not a real market. It is not a managed market, if by that we mean a market transparently operating yet in the context of regulatory groundrules (affecting providers, purchasers and consumers/citizens) which are consistent, stable and transparent. Health sector reform – or attempted reform – in other countries has embraced the idea of managed competition, but this is a very different animal, focusing as it does upon regulated choice of health plan by the citizen (Enthoven, 1988; Paton, 1996; Saltman and von Otter, 1992). The theory of managed competition sets out the principles for such regulation, to seek the benefits of competition yet avoid some of its pitfalls.

Managing the market in Britain, however, following the reforms has meant a pot-pourri of *ad hoc* activities: political determination of where new hospitals will be built; political veto of purchasers' decisions; and so forth. It would be better to call it 'political planning'; the language of the market was increasingly inapplicable and only maintained because analysts as well as managers seemed to assume it was *de rigeur*.

In the evident absence of a competitive market, the concept of contestability was mined from economics textbooks to seek to justify the new arrangements. (The then Chief Executive of the NHS, Duncan Nichol, used it in 1992.) Contestability is, however, a term describing (natural) markets with certain specific characteristics. To use it to describe Britain's post-reform NHS is to seek to impose precision upon an *ad hoc* administrative system. Competition is *ad hoc*, and is countermanded (when politically convenient or necessary) in an equally *ad hoc* manner.

Meanwhile, following this general picture of today's NHS, let us step back in time to remember the origins of the changes which have eventually produced today's heavily politicised and centralised service. In so doing, we will be reminded that the rhetoric of the time was very different, pointing to devolution of decision making and allegedly efficient markets. Instead, we have administrative complexity and fragmentation yet central control of objectives and rules.

2 Ideology, right-wing ideas and Conservative reforms: the Prime Minister's Review

THE SEEDS OF A RADICAL CONSERVATIVE RESPONSE

It was as a result of the increasing dissatisfaction in the mid to late 1980s with levels of funding, and therefore levels of service and equality of access, that alternatives to the NHS model began to have more currency. Before this, it had been a small, right-wing and 'libertarian' minority which had opposed the principles underpinning a publicly funded, publicly provided NHS. They had, however, been firmly out in the political cold, as had much of the Thatcherite wing of the Conservative Party prior to the defeat of Edward Heath in 1975.

There were fundamentally three options from which a right-wing attack on the principles of the NHS could choose. All of them started from the premise that popular demand for services outstripped existing supply. As a result, you could either spend more (but privately, it was now argued) or do more with the existing money. It is interesting to note in 1997 that neither of these has worked to any great extent. As a result, it is now argued that we must demand less from the NHS, we must ration and so forth. This has led the Right into a policy schizophrenia: we're spending too much, on one argument; but we're not spending enough, on another. In 1996, an article published by the National Institute for Economic and Social Research and a follow-up commentary by Anatole Kaletsky, the Economics Editor of *The Times*, exposed this contradiction (Flemming and Oppenheimer, 1996; Kaletsky, 1996).

For now, let us return to the three options around in the late 1980s. Firstly, removing universal public financing could lead to private financing, with possibly public insurance for the poorest in society, to be combined with privatised, or at least no longer state owned, hospitals on the provision side: thorough-going privatisation could occur. Secondly, significant user charges, meaning payments by the patient, could be instituted, ending the principle of the NHS as a free service. Thirdly, while public financing and even central financing could be retained, hospitals and providing units could be privatised or floated off such that provision, unlike financing, was no longer public. Options such as these were explored in the early days of the Prime Minister's Review.

Certain right-wing or pro-market critiques of the NHS, as just suggested, pointed not so much to the fact that it was inefficient and therefore by implication too expensive, but to the fact that it did not allow enough to be spent on health care. This inverted the Left's argument that other countries spent more and therefore more should be spent on the NHS. The right-wing version of this argument was that it was only in countries where health care was not provided through a national health service that more could be spent, as it was only in such systems that a plural system of financing, depending upon individual employer and state contributions to insurance policies, could ensure a higher level of spending. But this was itself a misconception. European countries which spend more on health care often spend more than Britain publicly, before one even considers the private. Sweden is an obvious example. But national health insurance systems such as in The Netherlands take statutory contributions from individuals, employers and the state. These are a form of taxation geared specifically to health, but some is claimed to be private spending by commentators who wish to suggest erroneously that Britain cannot afford to spend more publicly.

As in other areas of social spending, a significant plank of the anti-NHS argument has been that people will not finance the same level of expenditure on services from general taxation as they will spend directly on themselves. Such a perspective, of course, downplays the possibility that collectivised or socialised services may be more efficient, not less so. The overwhelming evidence concerning the NHS is that it is more efficient, and indeed in many cases more effective as well, than other systems.

There is also the alleged unwillingness of the better off to redistribute through the tax system and effectively subsidise poorer people's health care. However, given the sharp decline in the progressiveness of the tax system following the Chancellor's budgets of the late 1980s, even this stance is less tenable than before. The NHS model is a separate issue from the source of its finance. There is a good case that all individuals in the country can obtain better financial value from the NHS than from an alternative. Even in conditions of financial stringency, the NHS has continued to provide high-quality medical care for all, except where closures have denied particular services. It is the 'hotel' side of the business which has suffered most severely in terms of reputation, in an age when the population expects more than a no-frills service.

THE PRELUDE TO RIGHT-WING REFORMS

In 1979, Margaret Thatcher came to power as Prime Minister and Britain saw 18 years of Conservative government up to May 1997. Whether or not there has been a dismantling of the welfare state, there was widespread agreement even by the mid-1980s that the welfare state has been restructured (Taylor-Gooby, 1985). Until the end of 1987, it was not thought likely that the NHS would be restructured significantly, to accompany other changes in social policy. There are a number of reasons for this. It was one of the country's most popular institutions, as consistently borne out by opinion polling (MORI/Nuffield Provincial Hospitals Trust, 1985); only recently have shortages begun to affect attitudes to parts of the service. A national health service model of financing and providing health care is considered to be both equitable and economical. The government had no coherent idea of how to proceed with any radical reform, even were this desirable.

The essence of the NHS is that it is both publicly financed and, in the main, publicly provided. Public finance, mainly through direct taxation, allows central control of overall resources going to the service. Public provision allows, in theory at least, resource allocation to regions and below regions to be linked to plans for provision of facilities.

Earlier in the lifetime of the post-1979 Conservative administrations, interest had been shown in moving away from one or both of these principles. In the first Thatcher administration, the Secretary of State for Social Services, Patrick Jenkin, commissioned studies of alternative modes of financing and providing health care in Britain. In particular, he showed interest in lessons from the US and France. The tacit hypothesis at this stage was that a move to a system of national health insurance was being contemplated; since the aim was greater rather than less cost control, this idea was abandoned in 1982, by which time Norman Fowler had replaced Jenkin. Authoritative and politically neutral comparison such as that being developed for the Nuffield Trust publication *The Public/Private Mix for Health* (McLachlan and Maynard, 1982) had some influence in leading to its abandonment. Were a greater percentage of GDP to be desired for health care, moving to the American system might help (with the proviso that more of the financing would be private). This, however, was not the government's aim; quite the reverse.

The rhetorical claim that 'The NHS is safe in our hands' dominated Conservative statements between 1983 and 1987, dating from the general election of the earlier year. Despite difficulties caused by the level of overall finance and the fact that redistribution through the resource allocation (RAWP) formula was affecting in particular inner cities and teaching hospitals, the crisis had not yet hit, as it did late in 1987.

The crisis, partly real, partly media led, 'hit'. The government sought to seize the initiative by directing the debate from one about financing to one about provision and reform and instituted an internal review geared to exploring all possible options for restructuring or replacement of the NHS. The Prime Minister, say supporters and contributors to the review, was not intrinsically hostile to the NHS but was frustrated at receiving increasing abuse in proportion to what she saw as increasing financial commitment to the NHS. Agreeing implicitly with Enoch Powell's earlier warning, she saw the NHS's constituent professions as having a vested interest in denigrating the service, to get more money.

The review was to investigate ways of seeing tangible value for money. The Prime Minister saw the NHS as a black hole swallowing funds without trace or evidence of result. Although there was no immediate plan or conspiracy to dismantle the NHS, the government hoped to turn the crisis of underfunding in the opposite direction to that intended by those who plead most regularly that the NHS is underfunded.

ALTERNATIVE DIRECTIONS

The main advocacy for a full privatisation model, involving privatisation of financing of health care as well as the provision of health care, came from the Institute of Economic Affairs Health Unit, a component of a right-wing think-tank. However, the political costs as well as the financial costs of a privatisation of the sort advocated would have been high indeed.

The second major option – moving towards the introduction of significant user charges in health care while maintaining a publicly provided national health service – was also likely to be very unpopular politically. Naturally, the public, Conservative as well as Labour, would be set against it. Furthermore, pro-competitive enthusiasts such as John Redwood, then a frequent pamphleteer on health during the Prime Minister's Review (Redwood, 1988; Redwood and Letwin, 1988), opposed the idea of what they saw as a monopolistic, publicly owned service, charging its choiceless customers. After all, a pro-market ideology would call for competing suppliers to benefit the consumer, not a monopoly supplier holding the consumer to ransom. There were, of course, those who saw such a policy as being a vast encouragement to the private sector; after all, if one is having to pay for health care anyway, why not pay for personalised health care in the private sector? In this context, it was something of an irony to see the new Labour government, in 1997, refusing to deny outright their consideration of such an option.

The third overall direction identified – preserving public financing yet seeking competition in supply – gradually gained the upper hand during the Prime Minister's Review.

A disturbing aspect of the review was that the terms of its debate were set by individuals with little experience in health policy and management. This does not exclude them on the grounds of intelligence, but it did raise doubts about their suitability for conducting a detailed review about a complex service. The wisdom of the review was questioned by many close to the Prime Minister. The already massive managerial and structural changes set in train by the development of general management, if compounded by significant changes in the financing and provision of health services, would (it seemed) render the Service ungovernable.

More worrying was that the interesting potential in the NHS for the fruitful reconciliation of resource allocation and planning to meet need could be threatened by policies which fragmented either financing or planned provision. (This is not to idealise the NHS pre-reform. However, there were many promising aspects of NHS planning and resource allocation which were dismantled by the NHS reforms.)

What has been described as the 'silly season' of pamphleteering dominated the early stages of the review. Treating such proposals analytically, they fell into the following categories.

Firstly, there were proposals to end the NHS, move to a system of health insurance and return responsibility for buying care or insurance to the individual. These proposals would have led to more expensive, less efficient and less equitable health care. They were advocated most prominently by the Health Unit of the Institute of Economic Affairs (Green, 1986, 1988). John Redwood, former Head of the No.10 policy unit, also advocated *inter alia* radical privatisation (Redwood and Letwin, 1988). Less radical versions of this proposal also existed and included the significant extension of tax credits for private insurance. This would be inequitable; pressure for even lower taxes would stem from the acquired habit of purchasing expensive private care and would undermine even the rump NHS left behind.

Secondly, there was the proposal advocated in a number of policy areas, including education, to give health vouchers to individuals to buy care where they please, supplemented perhaps by private funds. This proposal could, if necessary, be combined with the third or fourth points below. Vouchers could mean privatisation of financing, as with the above, or a retention of public financing or a mixture.

Thirdly, there were proposals to float off the hospital sector and replace districts, as currently known, with health management units (HMUs), which would contract for care with public (now voluntary?) and private hospitals. This idea was promoted by the Adam Smith Institute (Butler and Pirie, 1988). It was a classic result of think-tankers burning the midnight oil to devise policy from abstract ideology. GPs would be associated through a contract with particular HMUs. Individuals might be able to choose which HMU to join, but referrals to hospitals by GPs would be controlled by the terms of their contracts with HMUs, acting like American HMOs.

This leads to consideration of the fourth proposal, to give budgets to GPs, who would then buy in care for their patients from the hospital and other sectors. The efficient and effective would allegedly prosper. The idea was adapted from the variant of the American HMO, which gives the primary decision-making role to a primary physician gatekeeper, who controls access to more expensive, specialised care and prevents unnecessary use. Professor Alan Maynard of York University was associated with this idea, but saw it as just that, not a finalised policy proposal (Bevan *et al.,* 1988).

As we move to the less drastic proposals, we find they tended to advocate retaining public finance, but encouraging more private provision. They also tended to retain the health authority rather than the individual as the direct purchaser of health care.

The best known proposal in this category was that of the internal market, proposed by Professor Alain Enthoven in his 1985 publication for the Nuffield Provincial Hospitals Trust (Enthoven, 1985). Dr David Owen's interest in this proposal, announced at the Institute of Health Services management conference at Coventry in 1985 (Owen, 1985), predated the Prime Minister's growing attraction to it by a number of years, let alone months. It was always likely to be a Tory policy, however, given its stress on markets. It tended to be viewed suspiciously by Labour due to its associations with the government after meetings of the No. 10 policy unit and editorial writers close to the Conservatives had embraced it, placing it alongside more partisan policies. Enthoven, while a pro-competitive analyst, was not intrinsically hostile to the NHS or a politically partisan actor in a British context. Indeed, to make the notion of the internal market more attractive to defenders of the NHS, it was briefly described as 'market socialism'.

The internal market, although better known as a theoretical slogan than as a practical proposal, would mean districts trading with each other to provide and consume care, with the roles of GP referrals and patient sovereignty unclear. It was at first suggested that the idea be introduced as a pilot project, although cross-charging between authorities existed already in an *ad hoc* manner in the NHS. It is also interesting to note that *integrated districts* would trade, in a market without a purchaser/provider split, in Enthoven's original model (Enthoven, 1985). Such a model does not entail by necessity any private provision, but was associated by the Conservative government with greater private provision, whether of clinical or support services. This would therefore include an external market, not only an internal market composed of public providers within the NHS.

There is a continuum, covering the above proposals, which runs from radical to less radical. But in all of them, the beneficial role of regions in strategically planning services and gearing them to equity and need in a wide catchment area would be lost.

The major advantage of the NHS is its capacity for needs-based planning. Many contributors to the Thatcher review advocated the abolition of regions on the grounds of abolishing bureaucracy, yet produced a system with higher administrative costs. Commentators wishing to abolish regions were not aware of their crucial role.

The review represented the heyday of Prime Ministerial government, when both the Cabinet and government departments were marginalised. The Prime Minister relied heavily on advice from favoured outsiders. A large-scale conspiracy theory concerning the government's intention to downgrade the NHS was maybe less convincing, as time passed, than a maelstrom of think-tankers opportunistically filling a vacuum. However, there were more radical ideas than radical thinkers floating around; we seemed to be witnessing the market principle undergoing a *reductio ad absurdum,* whereby alternative and inconsistent schemes were floated by the same authors to see which would sell. The tracts were not weighty, but the NHS was in danger of being weighed down by their implications. The heyday of the review represented the radical chic of the right-wing applied to health policy.

The main reform proposals which consciously built on the ideas of Enthoven came from the right wing of politics. The Left found itself understandably in a conservative role, defending the NHS from its opponents. When the radical Right had been marginalised in the 1960s and 1970s, it had been safer to criticise the NHS, from a left-wing viewpoint. But now such behaviour could be destabilising, to the advantage of the right.

There were also proposals in front of the review to change the system of finance for the NHS without removing its public nature. Both Conservative and Labour politicians made these proposals: the former Conservative Home Secretary, Leon Brittan, advocated a special health tax incorporating national insurance, thus promoting a compromise between the NHS model and national health insurance. Frank Field, Labour MP and then Chairman of the Social Services Select Committee (Social Security Minister ten years later, after 1997), advocated a similar proposal, although with less scope for private additions to public finance and less implication of private provision of care than in the Brittan proposal. John Moore, the Secretary of State in 1988, had an interest in tax credits for private health care to be extended beyond the then income limit of £8500 a year. This had existed since 1980, seen at the time as the best way of persuading amenable trade unions to enrol members. In the end, the Electrical, Electronic, Telecommunications and Plumbing Union (EETPU) was the main union at the time so to do.

THE STRUCTURE OF THE PRIME MINISTER'S REVIEW

The Prime Minister's Review, announced in January 1988, was so called because the Prime Minister announced a fundamental review into the future of the NHS in response to questions on the television programme *Panorama*, unknown in advance to ministers, civil servants or the Conservative Party.

The review process continued a trend in the Conservative administration of bypassing traditional policy-making bodies or investigatory mechanisms. Instead of departmental officials from the policy divisions of the Department of Health as well as the permanent secretary and others at the top of the office constituting the key personnel in the review, informal deliberations constituted the key sessions of the process, which were attended in the early stages by the Prime Minister and throughout by more informal advisers such as those in the No.10 policy unit, former members of that unit and members of think-tanks – the Centre for Policy Studies in particular, but also the Adam Smith Institute and, in the early days, the Institute of Economic Affairs Health Unit, before its prescriptions for dismembering the NHS's public financing system fell foul of an emerging pragmatism.

The review committee was formally chaired by the Prime Minister. Its other members were: Chancellor of the Exchequer, Nigel Lawson; Chief Secretary to the Treasury, John Major; Secretaries of State for Scotland and Wales, Malcolm Rifkind and Peter Walker; and Social Services Secretary and Minister of Health, John Moore and Tony Newton – the former later replaced by Health Secretary, Kenneth Clarke when the department was split at the end of July 1988. The civil servant leading the secretariat was Strachan Heppel, deputy secretary in social security. Economic advisers, permanent and seconded, in the department also contributed. There was no consultation on a formal basis with the British Medical Association, the Royal Colleges of Medicine, other health care professions' official bodies or the public. Invited contributions on an *ad hoc* basis from academics and others were considered.

The review originally was to report by the summer of 1988, but dispute over policy and difficulty in devising practical reform proposals prolonged its deliberations until early 1989, with the publication of the White Paper.

The review committee met weekly, with limited contributions from private health-care executives, businessmen, including Sir Roy Griffiths, at this time deputy chairman of the NHS management board and the PM's personal adviser, and generalists from the policy community on the right wing of politics.

In the end, the review adopted the core idea of provider markets within the NHS in an attempt to maintain public financing yet escape the bureaucratic system of planned provision. Some of the more right-wing advisers saw the review's conclusions as a half-way house to more thoroughgoing privatisation in a fourth Conservative term. The Prime Minister saw the NHS as a 'black hole', swallowing up resources without trace.

THE STAGES OF THE PRIME MINISTER'S REVIEW

It is important to remember the background to the review. Growing concern, expressed especially in 1985 and again towards the end of 1987, about underfunding of the NHS was occasioned by crises in large teaching hospitals, in London and Birmingham especially. The government felt increasingly on the defensive about the politics and financing of the NHS. The Prime Minister decided to move on to the offensive and announced a fundamental review on the future of the NHS at the beginning of 1988. The skill lay in transforming what had been a debate about whether funding was adequate or not into a debate about the nature of the delivery of health care. The review's conclusions were published on 1 February 1989 as the White Paper *Working for Patients*. By then, the debate had been transformed from one about the demand or financing side of health care into one about the efficient delivery of health care through provider markets.

How did this come about? Let us consider the evolution of the review. Apart from a brief investigation in 1981–82 of alternative systems of financing for health care, it was the first time since the introduction of the NHS in 1948 that radical alternatives to funding health care were being seriously considered in Britain.

The Secretary of State from 1987 to 1988, John Moore, was keen to examine alternative systems of financing: principally, various health insurance models ranging from national health insurance, publicly funded in the main, through to various alternatives in the realm of private insurance; vouchers earmarked for health care; and significant tax relief for private insurance.

The first stage of the review led to much pamphleteering by think-tanks such as the Institute of Economic Health Unit, the Centre for Policy Studies and the Adam Smith Institute (Butler and Pirie, 1988; Green, 1988; Redwood, 1988; Redwood and Letwin, 1988; Willetts and Goldsmith, 1988). These proposals were very general and concerned both the financing and provision of health care. In the end, Moore personally chose the option of a financing initiative, allowing individuals to contract out of the NHS on the analogy of contracting out of state pensions, a policy with which Strachan Heppel, deputy secretary in the DHSS heading the administration of the review, was identified. But such options were anathema to the Treasury as they meant unnecessary tax relief to those already with private insurance and, more importantly, the loss of direct revenue on a large scale, politically very risky.

Even Mrs Thatcher felt she could not move against the NHS and her personal advisers felt that the radical policy agenda for the third term of office, including the controversial poll tax and various contentious privatisations, was already taking its toll on government energy and taxing public patience.

Given the deep political unpopularity of radical moves away from a tax-funded NHS, there was difficulty in designing proposals compatible with a radical review of the NHS within the bounds of political pragmatism. The Prime Minister's dissatisfaction with Moore's radical yet impractical proposals on the financing side, yet absence of ideas concerning the provision of health care on the supply side, led to his dismissal in July 1988 from the Department of Health half of his job, and later to complete dismissal in 1989. The department was now split into two sections, health and social security.

Phase two of the review was marked by consolidation by the new Secretary of State for Health, Kenneth Clarke, formerly Minister of State in the Department from 1982 to 1985. Clarke, a supporter of the NHS when set against many of his more sceptical Conservative colleagues, was thought likely to abandon radical ideas altogether and to go further down the road of strengthening public management, as represented by the Griffiths Inquiry in 1983 (Griffiths, 1983) with which he (rather than the Secretary of State at the time, Norman Fowler) had been particularly identified. Thus, it was likely that existing initiatives for better management of public money, such as resource management and measures such as clinical audit, would be continued and beefed up. It was further thought that, as well as forcing doctors to take responsibility for speciality and departmental budgets in order to husband resources better, Clarke might seek to put NHS clinicians on short-term contracts in return for higher salaries. The rationale for this would be to make consultants more accountable to managers. In the end, their contracts were to be held by hospitals (trusts) rather than regions, as a means to the same end.

The review entered phase three when the Prime Minister's dissatisfaction with the lack of a radical agenda led to the adoption of radical ideas on the supply side of health care. The concept of provider markets, a broader version of Enthoven's concept of the internal market, became the linchpin of the review. Other less radical components of the review included further moves to medical audit and the control of family practitioner services. The move to a corporate management model for health care also was enhanced, as the NHS supervisory board, now wholly defunct, and the NHS management board were replaced with, respectively, an NHS policy board, composed primarily of ministers and businessmen, and an NHS executive, to be responsible for implementation of ministerial strategy (Department of Health, 1989a). More recent research has seen this as a move *away* from autonomous management of the NHS, distinct from politics (Klein, 1997).

It is possible to separate the management initiatives from the political, promarket components of the review. The essence of the reforms may be seen in retrospect to be a further move to tighter management, tighter control of doctors and workers and more rigid contracting for services from providers. Along with this goes the agenda of greater audit. There were signs even by 1990 that damage limitation required less emphasis on competitive markets and more on control by regions, and by the NHS management executive, of how quickly the new purchasers and providers could move. Regulation in the name of accountability to Parliament, and in particular the Public Accounts Committee, meant limitations on room for manoeuvre by free providers. After 1992, the market began to work, but (arguably) only temporarily (see Chapters 4 and 6).

FOLLOWING THE GRIFFITHS REPORT

The earlier Griffiths Report of 1983 had set out a blueprint which would take politics out of the NHS and provide a corporate management board, as in nationalised industries. The aim was that management could be left to manage. However, as the first chief executive and chairman of the NHS management board, Victor Paige, pointed out on resigning in frustration, this was never politically realistic.

The White Paper arrangements centralised political control and made NHS management, from the new management executive through to the more tightly managed regional and district health authorities, more likely to act at the behest of political priorities. A likely consequence of the White Paper's implementation was that political intervention in health care became more direct rather than less obtrusive, albeit in the context of a corporate management structure. Already, by the end of 1989, the ambulance dispute suggested that the NHS management executive was likely to act as a conduit for political directives, rather than as an autonomous management board.

These developments were an attempt to clear up some inconsistencies in the pre-White Paper NHS. A problem with the half-way house of the

Griffiths Report had been that the new managerial line of control from the Secretary of State and the NHS management board, through to regional and district general managers had cut across other lines of control. The Secretary of State also was at the top of a line linking regional chairmen and regional health authorities with district chairmen and district health authorities. The chief medical officer was the head of a medical line of control through regional down to district medical officers. A consequence of the 1989 White Paper was to diminish lines of control other than the key political/managerial one. Health authorities were no longer to be quasi-independent, drawing members from professional groups, public interest groups, trade unions and the public at large. Instead, they were to be effectively corporate boards.

Thus, health authorities would no longer be loosely representative bodies rooted in their communities, but mere adjuncts to their local management boards. Alternative sources of advice to the Department of Health, whether through lay authorities or through the medical professions, were to be subjugated to the new structures, entrenching general management, which established firm lines of control from the top down. The irony here is that political unpopularity deriving from rationalising measures, such as hospital closures, was not deflected to the locally responsible managers, as ministers hoped, but channelled upwards to ministers, who were no longer protected by independent-minded health authorities.

A publicly funded NHS, whether or not services are publicly provided, is bound to be scrutinised by Parliament and government. The difficulty in devising a management board which, in the original Griffiths Report, was allegedly to be independent of the Department of Health was that parliamentary and government oversight might be reduced. Ministers were never likely to loosen the reins to this extent; otherwise, they would be left with responsibility without power to act.

The White Paper's attempts at furthering the general management of the NHS lay in a different direction. They accepted political control and that the new policy board would be dominated by politicians as well as industrialists. The management executive would be the management arm for the policy board, shorn of the pretensions which the original NHS management board originally had, and the absence of which in practice led to the resignation of Victor Paige in 1986, that it would be independent, rather like the board of a fairly autonomous public corporation.

In his Rock Carling monograph, Sir Kenneth Stowe, former permanent secretary of the DHSS, argued that most change in the NHS has foundered on the rocks of the need for public monitoring and public control, by the Public Accounts Committee, indirectly in recent years by the Social Services Select Committee or, indeed, by the Health Services Commissioner, the ombudsman (Stowe, 1988).

THE CONTENTS OF THE WHITE PAPER

The eight Working Papers which followed the White Paper after two weeks (with more to follow) did not provide much more detail than the Paper itself. The key themes of the White Paper are reflected in the titles of the Working Papers, which are only marginally amended in the following list, of which the first three are the most radical and crucial.

1. Self-Governing Hospitals (later to be all providers)
2. Funding and Contracts for Hospital Services
3. Practice Budgets for GPs
4. Indicative Prescribing Budgets for GPs
5. Capital Charges
6. Medical Audit
7. NHS Consultants: Appointments, Contracts, and Awards
8. Implications for Family Practitioner Committees (Department of Health, 1989b)

Self-Governing Hospitals

The most plausible rationale for self-governing hospitals is to free up providing institutions to compete as flexible actors in the marketplace. For the purposes of this theory, hospitals are to include all forms of health care. Secretary of State Kenneth Clarke announced later in 1989, under some pressure, that community units, or parts of them, would also be allowed (later forced) to opt out. As in education, the ideology argues that independent institutions are more able to set their own objectives and to manage their own resources and then make themselves appealing to the client, whether this is the parent, in education, or the sick person's advocate, in the NHS – the health manager acting as purchaser of health care.

The irony is that where competition looked likely to work and to force closures in, say, London, the government halted trust status for hospitals seeking it in October 1991 in order to set up the Tomlinson Commission to plan London's future. Only where trusts could be guaranteed survival were they allowed, at first. Later, all providers became trusts, even when local communities were opposed, as they always were. In some early 'test cases' – most prominently Guy's Hospital in London – local consultation was narrowed by the government, acting through the NHS management executive, to mean the hospital's doctors. Carrots and sticks were then applied (BBC *Public Eye*, 1996).

The policy of making trust status voluntary at first was probably a mistake. It was, however, based less on a desire to appear democratic (although this counted, before but not after the 1992 general election) than on a fear that many hospitals could not cope with self-governing status. When the policy became universal, it was accompanied by central control of the agenda, and of providers, to a much greater extent than originally envisaged. Making all providers statutorily established trusts has, however, made closures and mergers more difficult (as local boards have to be appeased) and thus adversely affected the Conservatives' later objectives. They became a victim of the fragmentation which they had thought would be useful in thwarting 'socialist planning'.

Contracting for Services

Funding and provision were now, in theory, separated. The district was now the purchaser, having been given funds by the Department of Health via the region. Contracts with providers, whether self-governing hospitals and units or directly managed units, were now made by the district, which determined the mix of services to be provided.

In practice, however, this measure may have robbed the NHS of a considerable amount of flexibility. For the difficulties inherent in predicting and costing need for health care, when quantified by a system of contracts, have produced a more bureaucratic and regulated NHS than existed prior to the White Paper. Health authorities (which replaced the earlier districts in 1996 and now included primary care as well) are the purchasers of health care for their residents. Thus, patients and GPs have their preferences subjugated to those of managers.

Pre-reforms, GP referral was not controlled, even if the money did not always follow the patient quickly because of the operation of the resource allocation formula. Post-reforms, although the money follows the patient, with units paid in proportion to their workload, referrals are rationed. This will be done rationally in the eyes of the White Paper's defenders, by managers. The age of a rationed NHS, long existing informally, has formally dawned. Waiting lists are the responsibility of the purchaser in such a system. It is politically convenient to cut waiting lists simply by not allowing people on to them. Pretending that rationing can be done by scientific criteria which are both intellectually robust and morally acceptable, or either, is a deceit.

The policy of charging for capital (Department of Health, 1989b) meant logically that regions would be the bankers which provide hospitals and units with capital or deny them. Capital charging is intended to ensure that prices of services reflect capital costs – depreciation and rental of capital, on accounting principles – that is, that costs are global, as in the private sector, where any purchase generally reflects the total cost of production and not just the running costs. Making the region the disburser of capital, on the provision side, was thought necessary, since the district was the purchaser on the demand side.

Later, however, regions were abolished (in 1996); all providers had become trusts (most by 1993–94) and public capital dried up. In this environment, capital charging was either made directly by private suppliers of (expensive) capital or expected to be found from providers' rate of return on capital, in practice an extra squeeze on costs. Where capital was private, as with the Private Finance Initiative, which was applied to the NHS as elsewhere in the public sector, providers had to sign long-term deals with the private companies which provided it. This interfered with contracting (in one case, a contract of 25 years was required). It also led to the postponement of short-term costs, but at the cost of big bills in the future, as profit-taking private suppliers of capital expected a higher rate of return than on public capital. The latter, however, was ruled out politically, where possible, in order to cut taxes for electoral reasons and also in order to satisfy the Treasury's peculiar convention that all public investment was a negative call on the Public Sector Borrowing Requirement and therefore a 'bad' rather than a 'good' (which it might be in reality).

Furthermore, central control by the politicians of the capital agenda has meant that even detailed decisions about priorities for new capital have been centralised. Bureaucracy and delays have also hamstrung the Private Finance Initiative, which had become an embarrassment by the 1997 general election and the source of a lead item on BBC2's *Newsnight*. A number of new pieces of legislation have been necessary, including the diminution of risk to private partners and, at the time of writing, major Private Finance Initiative schemes have run into the ground because private partners have been wary of signing deals with NHS trusts which have dubious financial status in law. In the absence of public capital, the Labour government ironically extended the PFI.

IMPLEMENTATION

The problem was that the Department of Health defined the success of the White Paper in terms of process – how many hospitals opt out, how contracts are drawn up – rather than outcomes defined by the criterion of how far the health status of a target population is improved.

A major danger is that regulating competition is a much more bureaucratic and cumbersome exercise than merely running a planned public health service. This may go against the prevailing political rhetoric but is a lesson which we would do well to absorb from the US. Protecting the needs of untrendy local services and poorer local populations and groups is a major challenge following the review and White Paper.

The internal market was originally suggested by Enthoven as a means of solving the problems faced by large teaching hospitals which were losing money under the RAWP formula: gaining districts (purchasers) outside London could buy services from losing districts' hospitals, allowing, for example, London teaching hospitals to be rewarded for work done for other districts. The essence of Enthoven's idea was to ensure that workload was adequately rewarded. The RAWP formula had in fact sought to provide funds to compensate districts for work done for other districts. Indeed, in certain circumstances it could benefit districts' targets, if not their current allocation, to concentrate on work for other districts. For such crossboundary flows were costed at national average cost and if a district's target for its residents was low, then this might be a good way, in theory, of boosting targets. The problem was that it was only a possibly far-off target that benefited, not current allocation. Furthermore, if district A benefited by having its target so adjusted for treating district B's residents, district B could continue what would become a beggar-my-neighbour policy by treating A's patients. Additionally, poor costing meant that districts could not know if particular referred patients would cost more or less than their average costs, even if GPs and hospital doctors were willing to implement theoretical management games!

The formula reimbursed districts for work for other districts only indirectly and slowly. Ironically, given its origins in helping London by allowing its hospitals to charge, the White Paper may now herald the closure of expensive London services, other than those in self-governing hospitals, and a move of provision to the provinces which was ironically never achieved by direct planning in the 1960s and 1970s. This is because districts outside London may eschew London's services on the grounds of cost. Enthoven's assumption that the quality of services in London would save them may not be realised.

Progressing by means of pilot projects was advocated by Enthoven and this advice was not taken by the government. In defence of the government at the time, it can be argued that the opting out of hospitals, which occurs gradually, and the gradual evolution of practice budgets for some general practices in effect take the form of pilot projects. However, the political need to make things succeed prevented scientific assessment of developments, as extra money was pumped in to prevent the failure of showpiece initiatives such as new self-governing trust hospitals and GP fundholders. Political pressure ensured that interest was expressed in becoming a trust, without intellectual or analytical consideration, by many hospitals and units. The fragmentation of formerly cohesive hospital and community units was accepted at a stroke, reversing years of slow but fruitful planning. Devolution in itself is not necessarily a virtue.

The rationing of health care at the point of purchase by a global purchaser, rather than allowing rationing to be done informally by providers of care, is the key theme of the White Paper. However, the status of the district health authority as a monopsonistic public purchaser was diluted by giving optional budgets to GPs for certain categories of non-immediate hospital care. This policy was opposed by many involved in the NHS review. In the end it slipped in, supported by those, primarily the Prime Minister, who liked the sound of pluralism in financing without necessarily thinking through the consequences. Later, GP fund-holding was extended (see Chapters 3 and 4). After the 1997 elections, the Labour government retained the idea of rationing by purchaser; indeed, they devolved the responsibility to locality groupings where possible, below the level of the health authority.

THE POLITICS OF THE WHITE PAPER

Politically, the White Paper can be seen as a clever exercise in diverting attention from the underfunding of the NHS by international standards (BMA, 1988, 1989).

Underfunding occurs despite the fact that, also by international standards, the NHS is extremely efficient and effective at producing health outcomes from limited amounts of money. It is of course a contentious debate as to how much the health status of a country's population is related to its health service. There are those who point to the fact that differences in health status between social classes are as wide now as they were at the foundation of the NHS. The complexity of such debates apart, a good case can be made that the NHS has ameliorated what would have been an even worse situation.

The essence of the reforms has been to focus attention upon the provision and management of health care. It is hoped that by decentralising responsibility for provision to hospitals and units, the buck can be passed as regards adequacy and quality of service. Within hospitals, the buck can be passed to clinical directors within specialties.

The response of most doctors was predictable. It was unfortunate for both the Secretary of State and the doctors that the debate about the White Paper in general became confused with the debate about the new contract for GPs. Doctors' fears as to professional autonomy and levels of remuneration were accompanied by a genuine fear that the benefits of a publicly planned NHS – which they have come to accept enthusiastically, however slowly – are in danger of being lost as a result of the White Paper. Much argument against the White Paper by clinicians and GPs has often been rooted in an altruistic defence of the service. The heat of the battle was exemplified by the BMA's poster campaign after the 1989 launch of the White Paper: 'What do you call a man who won't take medical advice? Mr Clarke' and 'How can it be a local anaesthetic when the hospital's 50 miles away?'. Kenneth Clarke, never the shrinking violet, responded at that year's Conservative Party conference by proclaiming 'What do you call a man who won't take medical advice?

Healthy!' and accusing doctors of reacting to a crisis by reaching for their wallets.

Hard-headed health service general managers, no longer the well-meaning but meddlesome lay administrators of the medical profession's rhetoric, became agents of central policy much more than they had been in the past. Health authorities and trusts became politicised in line with central government's wishes, as appointment of chairmen by the Secretary of State became much more dominated by party political considerations. General managers, soon to be renamed chief executives, were expected to be spokesmen for the health service 'corporations' which they directed and, in terms of loyalty, they were somewhat implausibly expected to combine the discretion of the civil servant with the evangelism of the private sector company director on behalf of ministerially defined health service objectives.

It is not surprising that the medical profession is on certain occasions both sceptical and obstructive when it comes to the implementation by managers of often ill thought out and politically motivated initiatives in the NHS, not least when these initiatives are given neither time nor resources to succeed before the next flavour of the month has taken over.

The NHS general manager was now partly a political appointment, expected to be 'one of us' in an increasingly politicised service, consistent with the then government's politicisation of public service. While there were significant and promising aspects of the White Paper, the politicised and ideological environment in which it was implemented held many dangers for a publicly planned health service, where resources were directed to those most in need. Ideologies and slogans were adopted from the language of competitive health care in the US which betrayed little knowledge of that country's mixed experience with competition. As in other areas of British public life, we have the irony that US-inspired competitive or privatisation initiatives were uncritically fostered. When William Waldegrave became Secretary of State for Health in 1990, he had to ask for 'business language' to be toned down; this was confusing for those eager managers who had been spending sleepless nights learning the new jargon.

It was the continual and recurring conflict between the pragmatists and such zealots which surfaced during the Prime Minister's Review. The right-wing think-tanks put forward radical ideas very much geared towards amending, if not replacing, the NHS, in the direction of both private financing and private provision. In the end, the public's strong belief in the NHS – and a number of severe difficulties in other policy areas – persuaded the Prime Minister that these think-tanks could not presently be risked with the comprehensive design of British health policy.

THE POLITICS OF THE BMA

During the debate in 1989 about the White Paper, Secretary of State Kenneth Clarke accused the BMA of always opposing radical change, whether that was the creation of the NHS and the debate leading up to it in the 1940s or what Clarke saw as improvement to the NHS for the 1990s. The charge is highly misleading. There is no doubt that in the 1940s the BMA represented some hostility by doctors to the proposed NHS. In this they were largely supported by significant elements of the Conservative Party. So what had changed? Had the Conservative Party suddenly become the defender of the NHS? Had the BMA, in the guise of defending the NHS, simply continued its alleged tradition of opposing meaningful and worthwhile reform?

The Conservative Party was always prepared to support private doctors in their fight to be free of government regulation, monitoring of contracts and monitoring of costs, as long as they were dealing with private patients not paid for substantially by the public purse. Once the NHS had been established and become both institutionalised and popular, Conservative governments, like Labour governments, found themselves paymasters of a publicly funded health care system. They were, therefore, interested in receiving value for money in this system. The medical profession, in turn, went from the position of opposition to the NHS to one of support for its social ideals, with, of course, some exceptions, while showing some natural caution and reluctance to be overmonitored and overregulated as to the cost and quality of services provided by doctors.

The irony is that, were we talking about the private sector, including private consumption of medical care, the Conservatives would in all likelihood have been firmly supporting the doctors in their desire not to be overregulated by schemes such as resource management, price controls and medical audit. The Conservative Party wants to limit public spending on health care and regulate the medical profession accordingly, while encouraging private care which can set its own standards.

Has the BMA been historically inconsistent? It has gradually changed its attitude, as has the medical profession as a whole. This is not to deny that there were some self-interested and overcautious reactions to both the White Paper and other health care initiatives. The BMA has its conservative side. Doctors will always over-oppose regulatory schemes which affect them, as with all professions. However, in portraying the BMA as opposing everything, Mr Clarke made selective use of the reality that the BMA's original opposition was to the NHS, while its opposition is currently geared to protecting the NHS.

The Conservative Party had undergone a more significant sea change. It was now leading the fight to regulate the medical profession, allegedly on behalf of the public interest but in fact acting upon a desire to divert the terms of debate about the NHS away from funding levels by comparison with the rest of Europe.

THE DANGERS OF THE WHITE PAPER

The advantage of the NHS, by international standards, has been its cost-effective public provision through planning. This was now in danger of being substantially lost. Even where intervention occurred, it would now be through cumbersome regulation rather than systematic planning.

For example, self-governing hospitals were not allowed to 'cross-subsidise ... to allow keener pricing of those services subject to competition' (Working Paper 1, p.11). This would presumably require detailed public interest regulation. Protecting local services also required cumbersome regulation, giving the lie to the idea that markets are more efficient and less bureaucratic. GP budgets, if subject to unforeseen pressure, were to be bailed out by district health authority contingency funds, as discussed in Working Paper 3 (Department of Health, 1989b). These required specially demarcated budgets, reducing flexibility. Furthermore, giving some GPs budgets for some hospital care diminished the money available for districts' contracts with hospitals, increasing financial shortfalls for hospitals, which could only be made up by their selling services to GP practices. This reduced the capacity for planning services based on awareness of long-term, stable demand.

Overall, the creation of a number of distinct, cash-limited budgets leads to cost shifting – in other words, to attempts at reducing expenditure by shifting costs on to another budget. If districts or GPs have contracts, for example, for limited numbers of outpatient consultations, there will be a temptation to shift some referrals to A&E. This is allegedly to be monitored, as stated in Working Paper 3, but the task is highly complex. GP referrals may have to be paid for out of GP budgets without the GP having advance knowledge of the likely cost. Working Paper 3 expected the GP to foresee all. Regulatory labyrinths were increasingly necessary to police the market.

There was no statement as to outcomes or improvements expected from the new policy; the government fell into the trap of judging success by achievement of mechanistic management targets rather than health service (health status) outcomes. The policy, moreover, was always likely to be subverted. In the arena of education policy, schools sometimes sought to opt out in order to subvert rational planning and avoid closure. Admittedly, while vigilance by the Department of Health could have stopped this happening in the health arena, a lot of managerial effort went into negotiations to obtain local and short-term financial advantage from the policy. The political agenda overtook any rational management of the policy.

In the long term, if self-governing hospitals succeeded in selling their services to private purchasers, whether individuals, firms on behalf of their employees or insurance groups acting as HMOs, then they might seek less and less of their core business from district health authorities or NHS GP practices. Trusts began to seek 'sweetheart' deals with insurance companies, such as Norwich Union in 1997.

There is little evidence from the US that, even when there are pressures to reduce costs, hospitals acting competitively are able to do so. This has applied even in recent years, when there has been an alleged glut of doctors in the US. There is anything but a glut in Britain; in fact, a main problem envisaged for the growth of the private sector is where the medical manpower and nursing manpower will come from. It can only come about through diminished supply of such manpower to the NHS, unless private medical education both takes off and expands quickly. That is why private hospitals or profitable NHS self-governing hospitals may bid up the salaries of doctors and the price of care, disadvantaging residual NHS institutions.

It was ironic to return the hospital sector – the whole system – to the unco-ordinated state of pre-1948. There was a good whiff of nostalgia in the reforms, despite their imagery of markets enhanced by high-tech corporate management. Government advisers openly interpreted their mission as being to restore pre-1974 autonomy to hospitals such as Guy's. It was also ironic to restore pre-1948 raggedness and absence of planning or rather, in the 1990s, absence of coherent as opposed to panic planning. To dub opponents of the White Paper nostalgic dreamers for 1948 was a travesty of the truth; fragmented provision and confused purchasing is hardly modern planning.

Apart from the rhetoric about markets, defenders of the White Paper talked of the need to ensure that money follows the patient, that workload is accompanied by reward. This is both reasonable and correct. Sometimes, bureaucratic means of trying to achieve this (the issue has not been ignored in the past) have been too slow or have had unintended side-effects. But it was perfectly possible to relate reward to workload through flexible planning, without the disruption of the reforms.

Central features of the NHS reforms

3

INTRODUCTION

The NHS and Community Care Act was passed in 1990, and the reforms started on 'D Day', April 1st 1991. Unwilling to be made to look an April Fool, Mrs Thatcher (before her replacement as Prime Minister in November 1990) had become worried that adequate managerial preparation for the reforms had not been made.

During the earlier review of the NHS, she had admittedly lost patience with the absence of radical ideas for reform. She thought others were stalling, including Kenneth Clarke, Secretary of State for Health since 1988. Now, however, the roles were surprisingly reversed. Clarke was ready to roll with the internal market and contracting on April 1st 1991, whereas Mrs Thatcher, who had had a sharp and disquieting encounter with members of the new NHS management executive in 1990, feared that chaos could ensue (Timmins, 1996). Given the advent of the 1992 general election, there was an imposed 'steady state' – allowing the reforms to 'take off' on time, yet using central command to order health authority purchasers to place contracts with providers which reflected existing activity and existing patterns of GP referrals. That is, the processes and institutions were to be implemented but the substance was to be delayed.

Since 1992, the sheer complexity of interreactions that have occurred as the various strands of the reforms have developed, at different paces and with different consequences throughout the country, has served to make evaluation even more difficult. There is, however, a need to understand the package of reforms and their effects as a whole (rather than to present critiques of how different parts are operating), in order to understand fundamental trends and their implications. In such a way the paradoxes and perverse incentives of the reforms can be more clearly identified and understood (Paton, 1995). Any reform process needs a continuing focus and clearly identified and co-ordinated objectives and it is not obvious that this is so for the NHS reforms.

WORKING FOR PATIENTS: THE REAL MEANING

The government White Paper, *Working for Patients* (Department of Health, 1989a) was distinctive by comparison with earlier White Papers which addressed major health service reforms. Its main focus was not only, as in the past, on structural or administrative reform but also on the introduction of the concept of the purchaser/provider split, with the aim of introducing a market system into health care. No standard organisational structures were at first prescribed for the relationship between different tiers and between district health authorities (DHAs) and provider units, although many 'reorganisations' occurred across the country. In particular, seeking and achieving trust status – managerial independence from their local district health authority for providers – absorbed huge quantities of managerial and political energy. When one reflects upon the heat (and little light) generated by hospitals 'consulting their local communities', which were invariably opposed to trust status, it seems clear that the government had made a rod for its own back. Although some hospitals' clinical staff eventually supported trust status, this was usually under the influence of ministerial and NHS executive sticks and carrots. Most prominent in the 'first wave' was Guy's Hospital, where Professor Ian (later Lord) McColl led the fight for trust status, opposed by Professor Harry Keen, who had been a proponent of the Resource Management Initiative and 'self-government' by clinicians but who saw the reforms as actually disrupting more effective managerial innovation (and in particular, replacing Guy's clinician-led management board with a 'lay' trust board).

The basis of the ideology underpinning the NHS reforms, and indeed the direction of reforms throughout the public sector, was that of the 'New Right', with its advocacy of markets for the production and distribution of goods and services. The concept of markets went hand in hand with the values of economic individualism and freedom from government which led to the unquestioning advocacy of privatisation. Yet unlike many other public sector reforms, there were no direct measures within the NHS reforms to introduce privatisation, other than tax relief for the elderly who took out private insurance.

Some measures could, however, be seen as paving the way for future privatisation, such as the giving of relative independence to provider units, and the subsequent Private Finance Initiative has been facilitated, at the very least, by the purchaser/provider split. More seriously, the PFI is a means of reducing allocations to the NHS and not just because capital is now privately supplied. Before the reforms, health authorities (which included providers) received both capital and revenue allocations. After the reforms, the theory was that one global allocation would go to purchasing health authorities (composed of what would have been both capital and revenue). Providers, now separate, would sell their services at prices which included the cost of capital, which they had to pay for through the new policy of capital charging. But in practice, purchasers were given 'earmarked' capital allocations (if any) which they gave directly to providers. It was the old system in new guise. Now, with the PFI, private suppliers of capital have to be paid back, with profit to boot. That is, purchasers have to buy services at prices which include capital and often expensive capital. But purchasers' allocations (capitation) do not include a capital component. It is not just that capital is allocated separately. It is now supplied privately but there is no allocation to cover the cost of paying it back. In the long term, services will have to be cut substantially to allow payback. In pre-reform language, the running cost (revenue) budget now has to cover capital as well, even for purchasers, who have to meet the costs of private capital in paying providers (who have to deal with their private 'partners'). This bombshell is as yet largely unnoticed and is only beginning to smoulder.

What is more, the cornerstone of the new 'purchasing' is the duty of purchasers to decide what to buy – and what not to buy – for their populations. Although this aspect was disguised from the public before 1992 and still is to some extent, the concepts underlying purchasing – prioritisation, rationing – logically spell the end of the road for a universal and fully comprehensive NHS. There have always been difficulties with this in practice, but giving up even the aspiration was a sea-change – and a spur to future growth in private spending, by those who could afford it, on excluded services.

A key influence on the reforms had, of course, been the book written by the American economist and 'policy and management guru' Alain Enthoven (1985), who had observed that there were no mechanisms within the NHS consistently to reward efficiency and high performance. The reforms, however, do not reflect Enthoven's vision, as in reform proposals in other countries such as The Netherlands, of competing health plans, vying directly for contracts from consumers or citizens. His British model was adapted to fit the realities of the NHS, at least in the short term. By 1993–94, Enthoven had distanced himself from the detail of the reforms (as well he might, since the detail was not his), although the then Secretary of State, Mrs Bottomley, consulted him about certain policy choices at a time when the reforms were at a crossroads. Greater consumer choice had not resulted and the fundamental choice was between competing purchasers (such as consortia of GP fundholders) and more 'top-down' regulation through charters and the like. In the end, the latter was chosen and further market forces, to give greater consumer choice within purchasing, were put on hold. Even now, the substantial development of GP fundholding (to a point at which more than 50% of GPs are fundholders and more and more of the budget for secondary care is available to fundholders) is not about more choice for the public so much as more pressure on hospitals and traditional community providers.

The heady rhetoric against 'provider domination' led to the purchaser/provider split, alongside the idea that providers should compete for contracts. This would give providers the financial incentive to cut costs and (allegedly) improve quality. Cash limited purchasers, in turn, would not only push for best value but would also seek to challenge both the clinical priorities of providers, allegedly dominated by clinicians to an illegitimate extent, and the means of delivering packages of care within particular specialties and indeed diseases. This latter area has developed into disease management and so-called 'managed care', under the rubric of clinical protocols.

The White Paper *Working for Patients* stated two objectives: to give patients, wherever they lived in the United Kingdom, better health care and greater choice of the services available; and greater satisfaction and rewards for those working in the NHS who successfully respond to local needs and preferences. It would be difficult to argue with 'motherhood and apple pie' such as this. One further aim, Klein (1991) says, was to challenge the status quo and force a re-examination of both clinical practices and patterns of organisation. To do this there would be a need to challenge medical power. Additionally, a challenge to organised labour was a persistent theme of the Thatcher governments.

This White Paper pointed to a sea-change in attitudes by NHS policy makers. It would bring in the potential for explicit rationing of care according to the priorities of purchasers, replacing the implicit rationing by providers after a process of free referral and making waiting lists the responsibility of the purchaser. Although the language of consumer choice was used extensively in the Paper, there was nothing in it actually to increase such choice, given the enhanced role of management in translating needs and priorities into contracts with providers. The White Paper was described in the first edition of this book as a potential tool for managers to 'enforce economy and reorientate employee relations throughout the NHS'.

THE PURCHASER/PROVIDER SPLIT – PANACEA OR PROBLEM?

Klein (1991) suggested that the real test of the reforms was the way that purchasing authorities were commissioning services and monitoring their delivery, crucial in determining what is being provided to whom, and changes in levels of service, access, availability and standards, over time. To this, however, might be added: is the 'new purchasing' essentially different from effective planning as was sought in the NHS without and before a market?

Our own investigations suggest that reshaping services has been carried out at a level higher than the health authority, let alone the GP fundholding practice, and that the new 'purchasing health authority' has been mostly just a mouthpiece for centrally stated 'government priorities'. All the management effort has gone into purchasing and contracting, yet it is higher level planning which is crucial in deciding just which providers will *exist* to contract with! The latter task has been downplayed in the NHS. This means that planning, which is still necessary, tends to be a frantic affair, conducted behind closed doors and without clear procedures. Converting hospitals into 'core' acute and 'community' hospitals, for example (as part of sub-regional rationalisation and reconfiguration), is still done by region and sanctioned by ministers. Yet there is no clear mechanism on the ground to carry out the process.

A common picture emerging from our case studies has been the marginalisation of the purchaser in service planning, squeezed between (often changing and even contradictory) government policy and provider autonomy, ironically as the result of the purchaser/provider split. Government policy has stressed, firstly, competition and then collaboration since 1992 – often, indeed, together! In Sheffield, for example, the two main hospital trusts (covering the Royal Hallamshire and the Northern General respectively) were at first forced to compete 'across the board' and then (more sensibly) encouraged to work with the purchaser in rationalising and sharing out services. During the former phase, the purchaser's search for co-operation was overridden by the then Minister of Health, Dr Brian Mawhinney. And even after the latter phase had dawned, a new 'pro-competitive' and opaque document from the NHS executive, *Local Freedoms, National Responsibilities* (NHS Executive, 1994) was used to challenge the new co-operative planning. One reason for the recurring desire to 'promote competition' was the characterisation of co-operation as 'monopoly'!

Later, in 1996, not least due to the growing salience of a possible major Private Finance Initiative in Sheffield, providers were encouraged to co-ordinate themselves, under a 'lead provider', to aid planning and rationalisation of services. Additionally, local purchasers (whose fragmentation and varying demands upon local providers had proved an administrative and managerial nightmare) were to be co-ordinated under a 'lead purchaser'.

Elsewhere in the country there have been swings between planning, maybe involving full-scale trust mergers, and competition as solutions to the problem of how best to rationalise and plan services for the future. London, Birmingham and Leeds are examples. Indeed the problem has often been that different strategies have coexisted. One chief executive of a specialist trust in London told us that either free and fair competition or transparent planning could have been good news for his institution; what was weakening its prospects was uncertainty and political interference with both competition and local collaboration by the then Secretary of State, in 1994.

In essence, providers were to do the service planning, the Department of Health's Executive would adjudicate on capital requirements (and possibly arrange the private finance) and purchasers would then buy the resulting services.

A cynic could easily say that such planning could be carried out much more easily without the paraphernalia of the purchaser/provider split and its ideological justification but practical redundancy. To return, after six years of the reforms, to the sort of planning that was increasingly sought in the old NHS, but now at much greater bureaucratic cost and with much more conflict and changing, indeed cyclical, assumptions (as well as changing personnel) – such did not suggest a new dawn of managerial efficiency and the realisation of the promise of the 'new public management'.

Another frequent character actor in our case study dramas has indeed been the 'lead provider', although often as the agent which subcontracts for services to other (subsidiary) providers, rather than (as in Sheffield) the co-ordinator of providers for planning purposes. This developed as a means of avoiding 'gaming', and even hostility between providers, developing as they faced each other as competitors. It is not just a case of hospitals contracting for associated or complementary services to other hospitals; community and hospital trusts also were often in direct competition, either to provide services (such as child health, psychiatry or minor surgery) or to be lead provider when the purchaser or central government sought that arrangement.

Again, fashions came and went; at first, lead providers were seen as an innovative market response. Then (in 1994–95) they were officially discouraged; government thought competition could be sharpened by forcing hospitals and community units to bid against each other for contracts. Now the picture is mixed. The question for evaluators is, of course, which models make most sense in achieving objectives in a cost-effective manner. Does contracting with lead providers, who subcontract with other providers, justify its transactions costs, which are high, in terms of services which are better than a direct planning process with directly managed providers could produce?

The evolution of health authorities into purchasers has been slow and difficult for many authorities, with many false starts in determining the basis upon which purchasing should be organised. Legislation in 1996 enabled DHAs and FHSAs to merge. Although described by the government as producing a 'single purchaser perspective', it has to be remembered that this has happened alongside the fragmentation of purchasing with the introduction of GP fundholders. The main move within health authorities has been away from purchasing by care groups towards locality purchasing, to be sensitive to the needs of smaller areas. But this diminishes the capacity to 'purchase' effectively and efficiently to meet populations' needs in an equitable manner.

A problem with local purchasing is that it may be bureaucratic and costly, yet productive of little or no extra benefit. Chapter 5 explores just what 'local purchasing' means and what it may hold for the future.

Another way to view the purchaser/provider split is to see it as the separation of policy from implementation or planning from management. When dealing with the large and expensive resource which hospitals represent, it is essential that there is planning on a district and a regional level, to ensure their optimum use. And separating planning and service management may actually be a mistake. As long as providers are funded in line with their workload, the public integrated model may be better than the public contract model (Hatcher, 1997).

If regions (and ministers) decide which hospitals are to close, merge and change role, why waste months of circular meetings seeking to persuade local purchasers and providers to adopt the inevitable?

It has only ever been a hope that by separating purchasing from the provision of services, a more systematic management of services would ensue and that resources would be allocated more efficiently. The cliché has been that purchasing is not 'yet' up to the job. Perhaps, however, it is the job itself that is suspect. To go further, the legitimacy of planning must be restored in improved form. Currently, planning is the covert necessity which occurs hastily but dare not speak its name.

THE MARKET – ROLES AND RELATIONSHIPS

The creation of markets in a traditionally planned health economy could only occur as the outcome of a policy change and new legislation. Centralisation is necessary to provide decentralisation, furthermore, in implementing such reform. Markets in any pure sense cannot be said to exist. In health, the market system has been variously referred to as a quasi-, 'internal' or a 'managed' market. It is possible that a managed market might bear a closer resemblance to a planned rather than a free market system.

Le Grand (1994) saw the NHS market as attempting to mimic a true market system and by its design, to try to achieve the benefits of better quality services, more efficient provision, greater user choice and more responsive services. It is not clearly understood that the so-called 'quasi-market' policy stimulates markets where they do not exist and is not primarily a policy to restrict markets for social or public purposes. The latter agenda exists, but is separate. Thus the confusion mounts.

The key question remains whether, in the provision of public services, a market system is appropriate at all and whether such mechanisms are directly transferable. It is less clear how markets will be able to cope with issues of equity and ever-increasing demand. The essence of a market system is the entrance and exit of organisations based on their level of efficiency. Given the huge costs of exit and entry in the provision particularly of acute health care, the feasibility of this ultimate test of the system is in question. To date, there has been little evidence of non-statutory providers entering the health-care market, nor are there any clear arrangements for 'market exit' for underperforming NHS provider organisations. Instead, planning still does the job.

Research by Ashburner *et al.* (1994) showed that an analysis of how markets operated required the analytical focus to shift towards the micro-politics of the organisation and the interorganisational network. Here is a basic contradiction, since markets undermine the collaboration that networks require. As a result, the market may create the *need* for new forms of organisational collaboration, while persistently undermining them.

The move towards a market-based system also has important implications for the management, structure, roles and relationships within the health service, as control mechanisms change, with traditional management by hierarchy giving way to a new-style management by contract.

The emergence of 'management by contract' can only ever be seen as a partial alternative to 'hierarchy and bureaucracy'. The fact that the NHS has always been a loosely integrated system of interacting organisations or sub-units needs to be acknowledged. The resulting requirement for co-operation and collaboration means that the importance of the existing network of relationships (which need to exist to sustain the operation of the NHS) has been given too little recognition or attention.

NEW TRUSTS AND HEALTH AUTHORITIES

The statutory structural changes within the 1990 NHS and Community Care Act affected the composition of health authorities and the creation of the new trust boards. These reforms attracted the least attention from commentators but were significant in that they lie at the strategic apex of the new organisations and have resulted in an increase in power in the hands of management, to the detriment of local authority (democratic) and professional representation.

To understand the impact of the changes, it is necessary briefly to consider the previous form of health authority and their role. Prior to 1990 the boards had undergone changes in their composition but had always comprised lay, professional and local authority representatives. No member of management was a member of the authority and the chief administrator attended solely in a reporting role. These bodies had been variously criticised as being ineffective due to role confusion (Day and Klein, 1987; Ranade, 1985) and having a lack of corporate identity (Lee and Mills, 1982), leading to the criticism that they were merely 'rubber stamps' (Best and Ham, 1989).

Not only was the composition completely revised but so was the remit for the members. The tripartite system of representation was replaced by a private sector board model. The size of the body was reduced to just 11 with five executives included for the first time. Gone were the professional and local authority representatives and the lay members became 'non-executive directors', also five in number. The chair was also a non-executive. Although there was no statutory requirement for anyone with a medical, nursing or health background to be on the boards of the new health authorities, the medical director and director of nursing had a statutory place on the boards of trusts. The FHSAs were slightly different, in that four of the five executive roles were health professionals, but acting in a personal rather than a representational role. To reinforce this increase in managerialist power, the new non-executive directors were sought from the board rooms of large private sector organisations (Ashburner, 1994; Ashburner and Cairncross, 1993).

The assumption appears to be that changing the composition of the authorities will increase their effectiveness but this cannot be substantiated. Changes to the composition of boards in themselves are not sufficient to ensure effectiveness. It is, however, crucial to consider the extent of a board's influence and thus their role and operations.

If it can be shown that these bodies have an increasing level of influence, then who is on the board becomes increasingly important. Not only is there likely to be conflict between the formal accountability to the Secretary of State and the acknowledged informal accountability to other groups and the local population, but the wide range of backgrounds of the old-style health authority members has been replaced by a more homogeneous group of people with strong management and private sector backgrounds.

Research on private sector boards suggests that there is little evidence that the model in use ensures effectiveness and clear evidence that, given the numerous scandals with Guinness, Maxwell and BCCI, there is little in this model to ensure probity. The private sector response was the Cadbury Code, which remains voluntary. Within the NHS the recommendations of the code have been followed and further guidelines issued to ensure probity.

One major reason is that with private sector practices in the NHS came certain private sector mores. Scandals in Wessex Region over the supply of information technology and in West Midlands Region over management services were instrumental in the adoption of codes of practice to seek to tame the genie newly released from the bottle. More generally, there was concern over sleaze and philistinism NHS style, satirised widely by comedians such as John Bird and John Fortune.

New solutions to new problems do not address the question of whether the new model adequately replaces the previous model, with its focus on accountability. The new health authorities and trusts are part of a growing number of non-elected bodies devised to run public services at a local level and responsible only to the minister concerned. The cost of policing both sides of the purchaser/provider split through such arrangements is considerable. Personnel alone is costly. But hidden costs of the complex new arrangements are bound to be greater. And, apart from financial accountability between providers and purchasers, there is a dearth of clarity concerning accountability more generally, in the new NHS (see Chapter 6).

The two key issues of membership and accountability are linked. NHS trusts form a large percentage (20%) of the new locally based quangos that have developed since 1979. As local accountability declines, the indirect control from central government has increased with the appointment of members. This is the so-called 'democratic deficit'. Although charged with responsibility for the provision of local services, there are no mechanisms to ensure local accountability and the previous broad base of membership has been removed and replaced by one with a narrow, private sector, managerial base. Such boards may operate in a more 'businesslike' manner but such a homogeneous group has meant the loss of the wide range of knowledge and perspectives with which to inform board policy and the decision-making process. Any moves to broaden the base of membership and to create a form of local accountability have been left to individual boards to instigate for themselves, and it has to be noted that many did recognise the need for this. Board composition can thus be seen as a key means by which the reforms have been implemented at all levels within the NHS, given the strong support for the reforms (and the ideology behind them) expressed by non-executives and especially chairs (Ashburner, 1994; Ashburner and Cairncross, 1993).

GP FUNDHOLDING – EVOLUTION OR REVOLUTION?

The emergence of GP fundholding has been referred to as the 'wild card' in the government reforms, possibly because of its potential for unseen consequences but more probably because by giving direct purchasing power to GPs, as independent contractors, there was greater potential for disruption to current patterns of health-care provision. (To those who believe in change by shock, of course, this may be an advantage.) The impact of GP fundholding, however, cannot be assessed without considering a range of reforms which were targeted specifically at the general practitioner.

There is doubt about precisely how GPs can facilitate the transference of services from secondary to primary care and exactly how the services will be organised and responsibilities organised. A speech by Stephen Dorrell, Secretary of State for Health, on October 18th 1995 to the National Association of Fundholding Practices annual conference saw the focus of attention moving, within the NHS, from the managerial to the future shape of primary and community health services. He saw the role of GP fundholding as being 'central and irreplaceable' in that process, ensuring an NHS that was patient centred.

The GP role had remained little changed from the 1960s to the 1980s. Family practitioner committees were then given autonomous status and independence from health authorities. In addition to their role in maintaining the patient register, administering the contracts for general practitioners, dentists, pharmacists and opticians, and paying contractors, they were given extra planning responsibilities. The objective was to strengthen their powers to ensure effective delivery of primary care. Independence was seen as a way of avoiding their needs being subsumed in those of the acute sector. However, the structure whereby all 90 FPCs were directly responsible to the Department of Health, with performance reviews only every five years, was seen as untenable in the long term. The extent to which FPCs took this opportunity to develop their planning role and manage primary care services varied considerably, with very few seeing it as proactively influencing the pattern of services. It formed the first stage of the process whereby the services provided by GPs, who were independent contractors, might be more directly influenced.

This was followed in 1987 by the White Paper *Promoting Better Health*, which introduced the concept of health promotion within general practice and used the proposed new GP contract as the means of implementation. The new contract was a key mechanism whereby FPCs could exercise their muscles in the management of primary care. The antagonism of GPs to the contract was clear: in a ballot conducted by the General Medical Services Committee of the BMA in July 1989, 75% voted against it. Nevertheless, it was brought in and practices had to face the reorganisation of services that it entailed. According to Bain (1991), the GPs' initial fears concerned increased workload, that the increase in administrative costs would not be met by the increase in income, and the feasibility of preventative clinics in dispersed and deprived areas.

In 1989, FPCs were renamed family health services authorities (FHSAs) and over the succeeding years, some operated jointly with health authorities. In 1996, they were merged into the new health authorities.

The introduction of GP fundholding can thus be seen, in one view, as a continuation of the process of extending the role of the GP, increasing the level of managerialism and introducing potential controls over the levels of expenditure.

In the early days of fundholding, in the absence of a formula for deciding the level of the budget, this was based upon existing expenditure levels and any unspent monies could be channelled into buildings or equipment and thus away from direct patient care. There are now moves to develop a formula for allocating resources to fundholders based on 'need'. Research which concluded in 1994, commissioned from York University, suggested that there was no obvious, robust formula. One of the major problems is the smaller size of population covered by fundholding practices and even consortia (groups) of practices. Another problem is the fact that fundholders may not hold the budget for all care. Thus formulae have to be ticklishly complicated, even if possible, to gauge need for specific (or partial) services across populations, while allocating globally to others, including health authorities. That is why existing levels of expenditure continue to be used. But they undermine a needs-based NHS where funds are allocated by formula, which has obtained since 1976 and the RAWP process. Only if fundholding is total and universal – and if fundholders are organised into large consortia – can these problems be considered. Then, of course, they are simply 'the next health authorities' but without representation of the public or broader interests.

Additionally, there is the separate issue of more equitable allocation of primary care funds *per se*, i.e. of the resources (currently demand led, not cash limited) for general medical services. Fundholding is a means of making global allocations which include this (and cash limit it). But there are other ways, as the December 1996 White Paper, *Primary Care: Delivering the Future*, described.

Keeley (1991) felt that the trend towards extending the role of the GP was to change the focus from providing services to individuals, towards organising the work of a team of health workers, deciding how money should be spent and keeping the expenditure within limits. He feels that to accept the role of controller of resources puts at risk the relationship with the patient who trusts that decisions will be made solely on the basis of medical need and not on principles such as 'distributive justice', which concern purchasers of health care for populations rather than individuals.

Another view of fundholding, which is more pessimistic, builds on this perspective and sees it as a new departure which threatens both equity and smooth planning of service provision. Such broader concerns about GP fundholding relate to its effect on the rest of the health service. The system has brought fundamental inequalities into the health service for patients, with different contracts held by GP fundholders when compared with non-fundholders (whose purchasing is carried out as before by the local health authority). Although this has initially meant that fundholders could get their patients seen ahead of non-fundholders, there is no reason why this should not work in reverse, should fundholding budgets be cut to control expenditure. The present study provides evidence of this emerging reality in certain locations. The system is thus inequitable unless generalised to all GPs and this would increase already high administrative costs to an unacceptable level.

It is important to recognise that the 'costs' of fundholding go beyond the practice and are incurred by providers who have to prepare individual invoices and letters to GPs, to ensure payment. The various forms of block and cost-per-case contracts between health authorities and providers are negotiated each year.

This has been criticised as making it impossible for providers to plan services in any comprehensive way or to plan for growth or contraction. How much more difficult is it, then, for hospitals to plan, when faced with innumerable GP contracts. GPs decide on care when faced with each individual patient and this is in fundamental contradiction to ascertaining health needs and ensuring equitable resource allocation for large populations.

In the context of a continuing squeeze on hospitals and the running of efficient hospitals by the 'price equals cost' policy, the policy of extending fundholding holds grave dangers.

Furthermore, given the need to 'rationalise' (i.e. plan) hospital provision, fundholding is not only a 'wild card' but arguably a source of costly anarchy. Its costs emerge graphically in our surveys and case studies.

Given that the extension of fundholding, both in terms of numbers of GPs and the range of services they can purchase, would add extra pressures on an already heavily administrative system, it is not clear where its future lies. Fundholders are beginning to form into consortia, to develop contracts on a larger scale and to take account of the health needs of the population and consider longer term development of services. If this were to continue there would be little difference in role between fundholders and health authorities and since it is unlikely that health authorities will be abolished, the running of two parallel systems would make little sense.

Several commentators have noted that one of the consequences of fundholding has been that it has acted as a catalyst for change. This has occurred both in its ability to move marginal business between hospitals and in their consequently being seen as key players by hospitals. Prior to the reforms, hospital consultants sometimes developed their services with inadequate regard for the needs or preferences of GPs but since the reforms, the balance of power within the medical profession has shifted, with GPs now being brought in to a more central role. This process may have been valuable in bringing all GPs into the commissioning process, but this feature is not dependent upon fundholding for its continuation. It may turn out that the greatest benefit of fundholding was its transient nature.

Additionally, 'giving power to GPs' is only as good a policy as the wisdom used to employ that power. Have GPs suddenly become saviours rather than villains?

THE WIDER POLICY CONTEXT

Primary Care

A foundation of current health policy is the catch-phrase of 'a primary care-led NHS'. Lower health-care costs have been associated with countries with a more highly developed system of primary care in the aggregate (Starfield, 1994). However, little is known about the relative cost effectiveness of providing care in different settings and by professionals with different types of training and even less about the health outcomes. A move towards primary care implies that there will be a substitution of some hospital care with primary care, but there is no evidence that increased primary provision results in reduced demand for secondary care. Furthermore, the policy currently means a crude squeeze on hospitals without the comfort of a national strategy for the acute sector (a persistent theme in our case studies and interviews). Without adequate investment in primary care and a maintenance of adequate hospital expenditure, the new policy could easily fall between two stools.

Is 'a primary care-led NHS' real primary care or merely secondary care outside hospitals, in the (probably mistaken) hope that this is cheaper? Such changes may not necessarily be cost effective or easy to implement. That few people appear to know exactly what the policy means for the NHS, or what mechanisms there are to ensure it is created, has not dimmed its apparent appeal on the basis of 'motherhood and apple pie'. One premise for the policy may be a counter to the acknowledged power base of acute units and their capacity to absorb NHS resources. There is a danger in seeing the move towards primary care-led services as a panacea to present ills within the NHS or as being basically 'anti-hospital'. Hospitals will continue to have an essential role to play and this needs to be assessed in terms other than targets for bed or hospital closures. The recent partial reversal of earlier projections for London should serve as a warning, as the King's Fund reconvenes its Working Party on London.

The ageing population, changing patterns of morbidity and the increasing capability of technology to treat more conditions have put an increased pressure on health service budgets. This rising demand for health care impacts initially on the primary care system, but its central importance lies not just in its gatekeeping role to acute care but in the level and range of care offered within its own remit. It is the foundation and first point of referral for a health-care system of increasing complexity. It is concerned not just with medical care but with a range of health-related services.

A key influence was the Health For All initiative from the WHO in 1977. By 1985, 38 regional targets had been adopted by member states against which they could monitor progress. From these stemmed six identifiable themes: equity; health promotion; community participation; multisectoral co-operation; primary health care; and inter-nation co-operation. Such a programme places heavy reliance on front-line practitioners and health professionals.

Current health service provision within the primary sector has GPs responsible for initial diagnosis, general personal treatment, referral to a specialist, health promotion and prevention. This latter role is shared by district community services, which also provide general and specialist home nursing. This leaves the specialist diagnosis and treatment in the acute sector.

The commitment to moving towards 'a primary care-led NHS' will place increasing pressure on primary care. As a consequence, Rathwell *et al.* (1995) have stressed that there is a need to examine the most appropriate ways of planning, organising, managing and financing primary health-care services. This will inevitably lead to a greater emphasis on 'shared care', where the responsibility for the patient is shared between different organisations.

This type of approach would suggest an increasing need for co-operation and collaboration, with the strengthening of networks, rather than competition as a basis for interorganisational relationships.

The implications of this policy statement have yet to be translated into specific policies for the development of primary care in the United Kingdom. The primary health-care sector appears to be at a crossroads with a number of possible futures. Given the number of factors which are driving the change, there are many varied developments occurring throughout the country, resulting in different institutions within the health service competing with each other. The lead may be taken variously by general practitioners, community services or hospitals with outreach services in the community. There is a need for a strong policy lead from the centre to forestall any possible confusion as to where responsibility for primary care development lies. By the end of 1996, a number of White Papers had been published – *The NHS: A Service With Ambitions*; *Primary Care: The Future – Choice and Opportunity* (leading to the NHS (Primary Care) Bill of 1996–97); and *Primary Care: Delivering the Future*. It could, however, be argued that these added to the pluralism of ideas and indeed uncertainty, rather than clarifying and establishing robust priorities. Ideas ranged from salaried GPs employed by trusts to supermarkets setting up clinics (later partially retracted under criticism from the BMA before the imminent general election). Predictably, 'private finance' loomed large. Again, as in 1989–91, it seemed to be a case of 'let a thousand flowers bloom'. The rhetoric now stressed consolidation, but the reality was rather different.

For example, if hospitals employed salaried GPs, would this eventually mean patient choice of 'health plans', as with health maintenance organisations – cutting out the public purchaser? That is, individuals would choose which organisations (embracing primary and secondary care) to join. Or would it mean direct funding of hospitals from the Department of Health, through its regional offices? If so, this would return the NHS virtually to 1948, with community services separate (which would incidentally also be a likely consequence of giving health budgets to local authorities, another old idea dressed up in new clothes in the 1990s).

EVOLVING TRENDS

Firstly, it is rarely the case that the money follows the patient, allegedly one of the great benefits of the reforms. The reasons for this are complex. To begin with, the statement itself was born more in political rhetoric than in a forward-looking analysis of the likely consequences of the reforms. The language of consumerism was used to justify an increasing stress upon markets and the whole panoply of the reforms. The already peculiar NHS market has been overshadowed in practice by a growing centralisation of objectives, enforced through the various agencies and 'quangos' of the new NHS. Simon Jenkins, the former editor of *The Times*, in his book *Accountable to None*, has pointed out that ruthless centralisation within the NHS is part of a general trend within the public sector (and even beyond, embracing what was always the uneasy territory of British civic culture below the level of national government). Rhetoric about decentralisation and 'local control' has masked the reality of market forces combined with central control. For example, the creation of trusts was justified by ministers as returning hospitals to their communities. This can now be greeted with scepticism, in retrospect.

Since 1997, the Labour government has begun to increase central controls in areas such as education and health, albeit without the ideology of the market.

Another reason why the money does not generally follow the patient is that the problem of alleged 'underfunding' remains. Again at the level of rhetoric, it was claimed that the incentives introduced through the market and the reforms generally would diminish shortages, somewhat contradicting the view that the reformed NHS would make rationing more overt. This was because the extra productivity would diminish the pressure. In practice, however, there is a strong sense of 'this is where we came in'. Sir Duncan Nichol, chief executive of the NHS executive (formerly the management board and then management executive), had claimed just before the 1992 general election that the internal market prevented the need for rationing. When speaking as an independent commentator in 1995 on the launch of Health Care 2000, an informal commission which he set up to examine the question of financing of health services, he painted a rather different picture. The 'underfunding' remained and the reforms had not altered the nature or size of the suppressed demand. (Hence the commission recommended proposals to generate extra finance outside public taxation.)

Plus ça change, plus c'est la même chose. In a context of 'underfunding', purchasers (or planners and resource allocators, in the old system prior to the reforms) have no option but to set aside block sums of money and seek to squeeze the maximum from providers once the latter have been allocated these sums. Contracting has become more specific and precise (some would say overspecific and overprecise) and as a result, the maximum workload has to be squeezed out of static sums of money (again, as in the old system, albeit in a rather different way).

Consequently, patients follow contracts and one can add to this certain perverse incentives. For example, it is a national regulatory policy that price equals cost in the NHS marketplace. As a result, increasingly efficient providers are reimbursed less for the same work. There is an 'efficiency trap', which means that more patients can only be treated by squeezing cost (which in practice means length of stay and, perhaps, reorganisation of provision). Thus, while purchasers wish more and more patients to be treated, providers can only cope, in certain circumstances, by restricting admissions and creating waiting lists (Adams, 1995).

The money may follow the patient if and when fundholders refer patients to their desired place of treatment and pay on a cost-per-case basis, up front. This was the phenomenon seen in early versions of fundholding, often generously funded by comparison with the rest of the referred caseload paid for under health authority contracts (although this was not exclusively the case) (Glennerster and Matsaganis, 1994). However, as fundholding comes to embrace more than half the population (although nothing like this in terms of share of the NHS budget), the situation is changing and it is fundholders who are increasingly having to make the hard choices themselves. In consequence, as they form consortia and become 'mini health authorities' at least for purchasing, patients have to follow their contracts also.

Secondly, anything resembling a functioning market (let alone the neo-classical economist's textbook picture of a perfect market) was the exception rather than the rule. Both analysis of our national questionnaires (conducted in two stages, in 1993–94 and 1995–96) and many of our case studies suggest that, while the institution of the purchaser/provider split naturally created changed behaviour, it was not in the direction of a recognisable market. This has implications for both the behaviour of providers and the allocation of resources. It also has implications for purchasers. Just what are purchasers up to or, as economists would ask, what is their 'objective function'? Providers allegedly compete for contracts. What drives purchasers? Are they the conscience of the NHS or is central diktat the stick which drives them?

Thirdly, the purchaser/provider split itself – allegedly the innovation which we can welcome – has significant costs and rather more intangible or variable benefits. These costs are not simply in terms of the resources required to run an institutional distinction between purchasers and providers at the devolved level which operates following the NHS reforms. (Arguably, prior to the reforms, there was an informal purchaser/provider split with the region as 'purchaser' and the district as manager of services for a catchment population i.e. a geographically based manager of providers as well as a more local planner of services.)

For the purchaser/provider split also creates certain types of behaviour and incentives, some of which are perverse (Paton, 1995). At the end of the day, as with the reforms overall, the question can be asked (although not easily answered!) as to whether the overall costs of the new arrangements are outweighed by the benefits. Even if, for example, the 'management costs' of the reforms mean that the total money available for patient care is less, it is still conceivable that the changes are worthwhile, if the combination of what economists would call allocative efficiency and technical efficiency (crudely, 'doing the right things' and 'doing things more productively') is greater than the costs of the new arrangements.

One can be generous and imply that – even if the total quantum of patient care is reduced, yet its appropriateness, quality or targeting is greater – it is still possible that it was worth it. Here value judgements inevitably enter. Quantity has to be traded off against quality. It may be that, in a 'democratic' National Health Service, citizens have the right to demand, if not always to expect, health care which 'experts' do not see as useful. 'Health gain' may be construed in a crude utilitarian sense, assuming we can agree about how to measure it in the first place, or it may have to be traded off against principles of equality (defined in terms of greater equalisation of health status) or equity (defined in various ways, principally in the NHS in terms of equality of opportunity of access to care for those at equal risk).

Another conclusion of our research is that purchasers hold increasing power, in the sense that they have increasingly tight financial control of providers. This is a two-edged sword. At the time of the creation of the purchaser/provider split, it was observed by proponents of the split that autonomous clinical practice (in providers) could be brought to heel by separating out the making of priorities from the carrying out of priorities through contracts with providers. This is, if you like, the conventional rationale for the purchaser/provider split and is a commonplace in the literature and in managerial comment.

Another side of the coin pointed out in the first edition of this book was, however, that institutionalising approaches to a purchaser/provider split might actually institutionalise provider power, not necessarily directly in the sense of old-fashioned clinical autonomy but in the sense of creating market power for providers who are now separated from a formerly integrated health authority. That is, providers of organisations would now be able to act on their own agenda where 'the market' or other aspects of the new environment allowed it. To some extent this has happened, and again some perverse incentives have flowed from it (Paton, 1995).

Over time, however, it has become clear that a number of factors give government and purchasers power over providers. There is an increasingly tight set of central policy imperatives which are translated through purchasers directly to providers. The purchaser/provider split has ironically become part of a hierarchy. Next, the increasing financial squeeze in hospitals (forcing 'efficiency savings' of 3% a year in revenue budgets and stringent capital controls) means that hospitals have to seek income from all quarters. Very few providers are in the position of being able to 'divide and rule' among their purchasers; they require all of them. Only the occasional provider (or certain providers in transitional situations) are able to take advantage of a pluralism in purchasing while maintaining adequate income. What this means from the economist's viewpoint, of course, is that the conditions of an adequate, let alone perfect, market are not satisfied. In down-to-earth terms, this means that hospitals require GP fundholders' income for basic viability rather than as an alternative source of income. Community trusts might be thought to benefit from such situations in terms of overall budgetary priorities, as their funds are now earmarked. The reality is however different. Community trusts are under threat from a different source: the increasing desire by fundholders to directly control (and even, where regulations permit or can be bent, to directly employ) the core staff of community providers. Thus community trusts' budgets are also squeezed.

Increasing central control of health management agenda means that local debates between purchasers and providers as to priorities are diminished in salience. It is important to be clear here about what is meant, for sometimes there seems to be an almost anarchic pluralism in terms of the conflict between purchasers and providers in different parts of the country. When one looks at the cold hard facts of policy priorities of budgetary allocations, however, it becomes clear that these 'debates' and conflicts are about structures, style and process. The mechanics of contracting and the haggling over payments, not something more strategic, are the stuff of purchaser/provider dialogue.

Purchasers have the power which flows from money, whereas providers have the power which flows from information. There is asymmetry in power between the two, on both dimensions. What this means in practice is that the purchaser/provider split can actually accentuate a position in which an increased 'turning of the screw' by the purchaser does not lead to more effective health services. Purchasers do not have information on outcomes or even on processes such as clinical protocols.

Another finding of our research is that there was a gulf between politicians and managers as to the nature of the market. As early as 1989, Kenneth Clarke made the statement that it was his opponents who talked about markets, not himself, as Secretary of State for Health! Managers in the early 1990s came to believe in the internal market just at the time that politicians were moving on to 'the next item on the agenda' and seeking to downplay the 'business language' about markets. Kenneth Clarke's successors, William Waldegrave, Virginia Bottomley and Stephen Dorrell, were all on record as cautioning about excessive use of 'market' and business language, which is of course quite ironical given the rationale for the NHS reforms. Frank Dobson's first act as Labour Secretary of State was to announce the abolition of the internal market.

Nevertheless, managers (especially but not exclusively on the provider side) have invested a lot of time and effort in seeking to create the institutions as well as a language to allow markets to operate. Most of this has been in good faith. It could be argued that the good faith has been betrayed and they have been left 'carrying the can' for costly mechanisms and institutions which are not justified by the benefits of markets (which by and large do not exist).

The final irony in this process is, of course, the political anxiety at the genuinely high costs of running a market, resulting in directives to all trusts to cut management costs by 5% (alongside other targets generally for reducing management costs). It would not be too cynical to suggest that managers have been encouraged to climb out to the end of the branch which has then been sawn off by the politicians. It is expensive to create the institutions of a market within a public service such as the NHS. It is ironical that managers are even indirectly blamed by politicians for a mushrooming bureaucracy which stems from a policy confusion, which is in danger of producing neither the benefits of the market nor the benefits of an alternative system born from integrated planning.

It is only fair to point out that the goal of the reforms, despite subsequent lurches in various directions, was always what economists call technical efficiency or greater productivity. The market was generally considered a means rather than an end. Even this general truth has, however, been challenged at times. At the end of 1994, the National Health Service executive produced a document entitled *Local Freedoms, National Responsibilities*, which set out a blueprint for creating market forces where they did not exist or restoring them where the operation of the market led to the gradual diminution of competitive forces. This is the old truth that very few markets – and certainly not health service markets – remain competitive. Whether one describes the alternative as monopoly or planned, rationalised services taking advantage of specialisation, economies of scale and appropriateness of location of services may become a matter of theology. Nevertheless, making the market an end in itself rather than a means to an end led to further policy confusion.

Where, for example, two hospitals compete in the marketplace and then end up specialising, the end product may be 'steady state' in which the local purchaser accepts the resulting configuration and works closely with both hospitals in succeeding years without expecting renewed competitive forces. There have been occasions, however, where the politicians have challenged this on the grounds that it is 'anticompetitive'. The case study of Sheffield suggests that a lot of time and management effort has been wasted because politicians cannot make up their minds whether the market is an end or a means.

A related observation which stems from our research is that while on one interpretation the market was a means of 'sharpening up' the general management system which followed the Griffiths Report in October 1983, it ironically became an administrative labyrinth whereby chasing the tail of the system's mechanics has edged out more strategic considerations. Since general management was intended to replace 'administration', administration of the contracting system as the 'be all and end all' is an ironic product of more than ten years of ongoing health sector reform. One graphic quote from the director of business development of a large united trust (acute and community) in the Midlands is instructive:

> I will quite openly say to you that contracting has gone totally and utterly out of control. We have got into a position where we have got spiralling requirements for information, spiralling requirements for

> dis-aggregation. More people are dealing with all of that sort of data day in and day out and it is a total and utter nonsense because we are counting, in the main, things that are totally meaningless. If you imagine that, if we add up all of our contacts in the community, we have got 750,000 contacts. Typically, somebody like a community nurse might do something like 20 contacts a day, they are all counted as one. One equals the next one, whereas that community nurse might be popping in for 5 minutes and putting someone's drops in their eyes, and the next contact is 2 hours discussing with a family issues to do with bereavement or going into hospital or whatever. Why do we bother counting that? What does that describe to us? It is totally and utterly useless and what we are trying to get away from with the GPFHs is get away from that and say what do you actually want your community nurses and community teams to be doing, not do you want to count contacts.

It is of course a challenge to move away from meaningless data and waste of management time. The problem sometimes is that the performance indicators commissioned and used by politicians require manipulation of such data in order to score local or national 'Brownie points'. The finished consultant episode (FCE) can be subjected to similar criticisms. Many of the performance indicators used to assemble league tables of trusts rely heavily on 'meaningless data'.

The term 'transactions costs' is borrowed from behavioural economics to explain the costs of conducting business through contractual processes rather than what the textbooks call administrative hierarchies. In the context of today's NHS, this phrase has virtually reached the newspapers, although of course it has to be carefully distinguished from management costs more generally. The data analysis within this project reinforces the belief that the transactions costs of both GP fundholding and of the 'short termist' market (including annual contracting) are high.

Ideally we would have liked to compare the costs of direct management in the 'old system' with the costs of producing services through market or contractual relationships in the 'new system'. This is virtually impossible, however, because of the constant reorganisation of the whole service of individual hospitals and of departments within them over the years, as well as a change in the nature of the business. As with other aspects of the research, what we can do is seek to paint increasingly accurate pictures of trends. An understanding of these trends can be useful in devising improved policy.

At one level this became a bipartisan issue. The NHS efficiency unit (which was part of the government-wide efficiency unit under the control of the then Deputy Prime Minister, Michael Heseltine) targeted extracontractual referrals as a source of unjustified bureaucracy out of proportion to 'the problem'. ECRs are of course an integral part of the NHS market as devised through the reforms; if referrals are made and care is delivered outside contracts, you automatically have an ECR. Abolishing them might be the easiest way to deal with the situation. This would, however, assume that all uncontracted referrals were paid or that none were paid or that purchasing became so refined that every possible referral was conceptualised and dealt with in advance! It soon becomes clear that none of these options is tenable, or rather only the first one is, but at the cost of undermining the institutions of the NHS reforms and in particular the system of overt purchasing rather than simply reimbursement of referred care.

The danger with 'targeting of problems' such as the ECR is that the old analogy of punching the balloon comes to mind: you solve one problem and one source of bureaucracy by creating another, as the balloon swells out at another place on the other side. There are signs, at the time of writing, that both the main political parties seek simply to displace bureaucratic costs based generally in the provider with bureaucratic systems of purchasing.

Prior to the NHS reforms, what happened to ECRs? This in itself shows a misunderstanding of the pre-reform NHS. ECRs could not happen. GPs (who, of course, did not hold their own purchasing budgets) referred patients and whether these patients were treated quickly or not depended on waiting lists and waiting times. The resource allocation formula sought (imperfectly and slowly) to reimburse care through referrals from one district or region to another – the so-called crossboundary flow. The problem inherent in this system was that, given the 'underfunding' at existing costs, there was often a discrepancy between the aggregate budget allocated indirectly for locally provided care and what was paid directly for care provided across boundaries.

Indeed, somewhat ironically, the system of provider markets was devised as one possible answer to this problem! It is therefore a 'coming full circle' that ECRs have become the bugbear of provider markets. It may be more sensible, or at least cost effective, to let GPs refer without disobeying contracts, i.e. replace specific contracting with more global service provision but to use (suitably managed) waiting lists as the language of priorities. Admittedly, this is less transparent, but it prevents overspecific contracts and the concomitant growth of ECRs, the tail that wags the dog in contracting. As long as services are funded in proportion to expected workload in the aggregate, adjustments can be made over time through the planning process. Seeking to abolish ECRs by anticipating them in advance is impossible and costly even were it not. The latter is in effect the old NHS, without prioritisation – simply replicating GPs' referrals in an expensive way through an inert contracting process. But seeking to abolish them by legislating in advance as to what will and will not be reimbursed is merely an invitation to 'gaming', i.e. reclassifying cases to get funding. Better to allow free referral (as in the old NHS) but improve systems of funding providers, so that efficiency traps are reduced.

Another suggestion arising from our research is that GP fundholders would increasingly commission in parallel with the health authority, but at high cost. Since April 1st 1996, GP fundholders as well as other GPs are 'accountable to' the new health authorities. It remains to be seen, even after Labour's victory, what the long-term consequences of this will be – the abolition of GP fundholding and integration with health authority commissioning, on the one hand, or looser regulation of a system with GP commissioning as its primary dynamic, on the other hand. Naturally political choices as well as simple evolutionary trends will determine these outcomes.

The Audit Commission suggested in 1995 that the benefits of GP fundholding in terms of changed service delivery were marginal and outweighed by both the costs of running the system and the dubious uses to which fundholding money has sometimes been put. It is also worth remembering at this point that the two-tier system, which occurs when GP fundholders are part but not a whole of the system, can work in the opposite way from that conventionally understood. As fundholders find their budgets squeezed, they may restrict referrals and, in certain specialities, in certain trusts, fundholders' patients may (whether or not at the behest of the referring fundholders) have lower rather than higher priority. Our research has uncovered this phenomenon.

The picture is, of course, very much a mixed one, with the opposite case still being more common. In July 1997, the new Secretary of State announced regulations to ensure *common* waiting lists for fundholders and non-fundholding GPs.

Another important outcome of our work suggests that there is severe conflict between 'market jostling' by providers and purchasers and the need for rationalisation of (especially) hospital services (in the light of a diminished budget for hospitals yet increased demand on their services). This demand comes from both emergencies and urgent cases and from 'waiting list initiatives' which is a leading example of an imperative which has been central to regional policy for purchasers and providers, as well as central to the internal operation of hospital trusts and their clinical directorates or departments.

The blunt fact is that rationalising services requires purchaser collaboration at the very least and, to diminish management costs, regional planning, to use an unfashionable term. A lot of time and effort has been wasted by encouraging providers to 'market themselves for anything and everything' despite the impending reality of regional reviews (such as the Birmingham review or the Black Country review in the West Midlands, let alone the London-wide reviews which are better known to the national media).

The final chapter of this book makes some proposals for ironing out some of the problems engendered by the NHS reforms, which might be termed 'reforming the reforms'. For now, it can be submitted that the main advantage brought by the reforms has probably been the possibility (if not reality) of more effective setting and meeting of targets for health-care provision. The main drawback has been the creation of perverse incentives, alongside a fragmentation of the service which is costly and also debilitating to the service in terms of its coherence and morale. This latter factor is intangible but sensible in the original meaning of the word.

The creation of more sharp sectional interests within the NHS has diminished the political resilience of the service as a whole and it is hardly a secret that this has been a deliberate policy on the part of some government decision makers.

Finally for now, intangible factors such as morale overlap with seemingly 'technical' economic matters. An important question concerns the cause of some of the increased productivity which undoubtedly has occurred in the last few years. It can be argued that rising NHS productivity is no different from previous decades. But if there is an extra cause to be explained, it is still an open question as to whether it is 'the market', tighter political and managerial control or greater intensification of work. Naturally, these factors may overlap in a complex manner. Important research remains to be done on longer working hours, intensification of labour and the 'reprofiling' of the workforce. They may be associated with both greater output and more stress for the NHS workforce. Work on accumulating GP stress is now becoming more focused. Similar work can be done for managers and certainly for low-paid manual workers, as well as for a whole range of professions. At the impressionistic level, one thing is clear: the contract culture is being used to 'squeeze surplus value' out of workforces within providers as well as the provider itself.

SUMMARY

To conclude this review, some key consequences of the reforms are as follows.

1. Competition between and contracting for services – with separate, autonomous trusts – may have led to specific financial saving in individual providers but at the cost of integrated care across providers. Additionally, overall costs may be greater, as a result of administrative costs beyond direct service costs as calculated by official statistics.

2. Supra-health authority planning – what would have been called regional planning in the old NHS – is still necessary but is now carried out less transparently and more bureaucratically, given that the institutions of the new NHS *per se* militate against it. Indeed, with the end of regional health authorities, such planning is now centralised.

   As a result, the Department of Health, or its divisions, make detailed decisions upon (for example) individual capital projects – the antithesis of the philosophy underlying, firstly, the Griffiths Inquiry and, secondly, the reforms.
3. 'Involving GPs in commissioning' is a *quid pro quo* for the loss of GPs' right to refer anywhere (except for fundholders – they of course have to trade off cost and choice, i.e. prioritising and rationing is devolved to fundholding GPs). Even this involvement, however, is misleading: service planning (the truth that dare not speak its name) is conducted at a higher level and 'GP involvement' concerns more mundane matters (See Chapter 5).
4. The costs of the reforms – embracing new institutions and processes associated with them – cover both investment and recurrent costs. Recouping these, as a result of political embarrassment at their extent, has been through downward pressure on service costs and also by arbitrary political diktat concerning reduction of management costs (costs which are, of course, a consequence of the reforms).
5. In most of our case studies and in a majority of the trusts and health authorities surveyed nationally, the purchaser/provider split and contracting are responsible for increased costs. That is, even if one discounts the market (where it is marginal or non-existent), the costs of running separate purchaser and provider institutions (and the costs associated with the contracting process) are salient. The idea that one can save a lot of money by 'abolishing the market yet preserving the purchaser/provider split' is therefore suspect.
6. Benefits from the reforms – desired and actual – required longer to develop. There is therefore the usual pattern, in large-scale organisational change, that costs are faster to appear than benefits. A major difficulty is one of attributing benefits to 'the reforms', as opposed to 'more money' or a whole range of wider factors.
7. Overall, the reforms represented another administrative reorganisation despite claims to the contrary. Wider consequences of the whole reform process, of a radical nature, cannot, however, be ruled out. They would be most likely to involve greater private finance of capital and a move towards more of a 'mixed economy' in health care in general. Trusts are already developing their own private insurance policies for individuals, for example. NHS hospitals *en masse* are marketing private care to insurance companies. Purchasers are drawing up more overt criteria for rationing. There is indecision as to whether

priorities are to be local or national. (This is a consequence of the 'purchaser/provider split' and of 'purchasing' *per se* in that, in the old NHS, services developed were in theory available to all. That is, priorities were *de facto* national.) Long-term care is less available on the NHS, with Labour having a Royal Commission to look at this.

4 The market, the purchaser/provider split and contracting: surveys and case studies

INTRODUCTION

Following the reforms, both hospital and community units (trusts) have experienced significant change in both the organisation and provision of health-care services. Not only have they been engaged in their primary work of providing health-care services but they have had to respond and adapt to a range of policy issues – junior doctors' hours, the Patient's Charter, waiting times initiatives and the development of a 'primary care-led NHS' – as well as the major challenge: implementing the changes arising from *Working for Patients*.

The latter have included greater managerial autonomy (as units attained trust status); the development of internal accounting and information systems in order to provide crucial support to their new roles in the market; and changes in organisational culture affecting both managers and clinicians. Correspondingly, the role and organisation of health authorities (HAs) as purchasers have also witnessed considerable transformation.

A major part of our research consisted of a quantitative investigation. This consisted of two stages. The first, smaller survey in early 1994 aimed to investigate the relationship between purchasers and providers and the nature of competition. Questionnaires were sent to all trusts and health authorities and a sample of general practice fundholders (GPFHs) in England and Wales.

The second, more intensive, survey took place in late 1995–early 1996 and concentrated specifically on all (provider) trusts (acute, community and combined) and all (purchaser) HAs in England. This was, in some respects, a follow-on from the first survey, but also went on to emphasise the issue of transactions costs, particularly in respect of marketing, contracting and monitoring.

Both surveys acted as a framework for, and basis for choice of, a series of in-depth case studies of providers, purchasers and regions, and provided information on marketing, contracting and monitoring as well as relationships in general between providers and purchasers (both HAs and GPFHs). The second survey sought a wider range of more complex information from trusts and HAs. Data presented below come from the second survey unless otherwise stated.

INCOME: MARKETS OR LOCALISM?

The median HA budget (in the second survey) was £182m (Figure 4.1). Size of budget was highly correlated with the number of staff (whole time equivalents) (WTE) employed by the HAs ($r = 0.45$, $p < 0.05$). The median number of WTEs was 96 although a quarter had more than 150 and 12% 55 or less.

Eighty-one percent of HAs had the majority of their budget allocated to hospital acute care while percentages for primary care ranged from less than 1% to 48%. Figure 4.2 shows the 'typical' allocation of an HA's budget based on the mean.

Twelve HAs stated there had already been a shift towards primary and community care in the previous three years in how their budget was allocated.

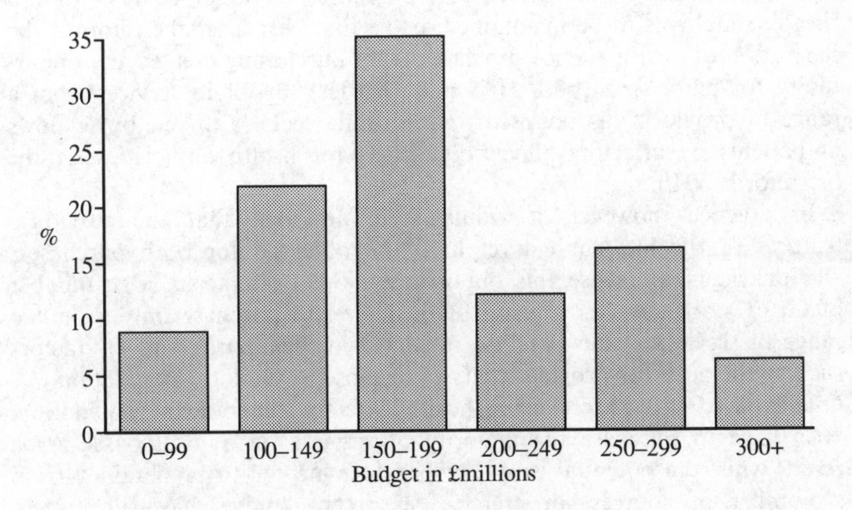

Figure 4.1. Size of health authority budgets in 1994–95.

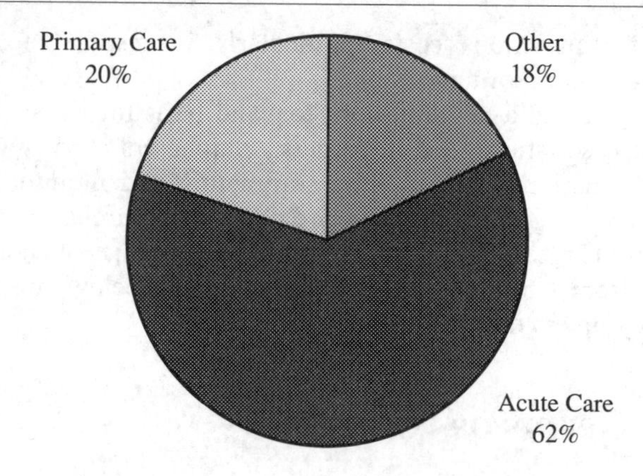

Figure 4.2. How the typical HA's budget is allocated

When asked how they felt this would change over the next three years, 20 HAs said there would be a shift (or a further shift) from acute services towards primary or community care.

The NHS market, apart from setting up a competitive environment for providers, created (in theory at least) a market in which providers could shop around for purchasers. In other words, following the reforms, provider units were not tied to their local HA for funding (apart from 'cross boundary flows' of money for patients from outside) but could seek the custom of any health-care purchasers. And of course, while a 'steady state' was to be maintained in the first year after the reforms, the separation of health service provision from purchasing created the opportunity for purchasers (both HAs and GPFHs) to obtain services from a range of providers, as opposed to a formula seeking to reimburse flows of patients by affecting allocation targets for health authorities, in the pre-reform NHS.

In practice, however, it would seem apparent that the structural features of the internal market limit the potential for both purchasers and providers to realise this opportunity. For example, a large number of GPFHs are able, as a result of their size, to purchase only a limited range of services, while HAs are restricted in their purchasing by factors such as the need for provider units to be close to the local population.

That is to say, in procuring health care for the resident population, HAs have to purchase the majority of services on a local basis. As a result, while the potential exists for provider income to be obtained from a number of sources, in practice, as recent studies have illustrated, the majority of trusts remain heavily reliant on their local HA for the majority of their income (NAHAT, 1994). This locality issue becomes evident in the answers to our surveys.

There have been some changes in the proportion of income derived from different sources by providers during the past few years. The NAHAT study in 1994 (NAHAT, 1994) highlighted that income from all HAs fell from 92% of total income in 1992–93 to a forecast 86% in 1994–95. This fall in HA income was accompanied by a general increase in the proportion of income obtained from GPFHs from 2% in 1992–93 to 6% in 1994–95. This pattern of dependence was similarly evident in our project.

The extension of GP fundholding up to 1997 will, of course, have significantly increased the amount of provider income from this source. There are now 'total fundholders' who purchase all care (as well as providing their own primary care from this global budget); 'standard fundholders' who purchase non-urgent and less expensive secondary care; and first-level fundholders, who hold their own budget for primary and community care. Additionally, there are larger consortia of fundholders set up (as well as those evolving through local mergers) to cover whole geographical areas – say, a third of a health authority's area.

Information was requested from providers regarding the composition of their income from different sources – such as the host HA, non-local HAs and GPFHs – to discover whether trusts were dependent on a few local purchasers for their income or whether, with the establishment of the 'internal market', trusts' income was derived from a number of purchasers. While all trusts indicated that their income was derived from a number of different purchasers, for the majority of trusts their income was still dominated by the host HA. However the overall dominance of HAs would appear to be declining if one considers the results of this project alongside an earlier study conducted by NAHAT (although it should be remembered that the two cohorts are not coterminous). In 1992–93, for example, 63% of providers obtained between 90% and 100% of their income from local health authorities and 95% obtained between 80% and 100%. By 1994–95 only 35% obtained between 90% and 100% and three quarters 80–100% (NAHAT, 1994). This pattern of decline in the overall income obtained from HAs was again apparent when comparing such results with the data from the current project. Only 8% of trusts indicated that they received 90–100% of their income from their local HA, with 31% reporting that the local HA income accounted for 80–100%.

However, the dominance of the local HA as the primary purchaser remained strong in that the majority of trusts (64%) indicated that such funding accounted for 70% or more of their annual income. A major tenet of the market is therefore missing – that pluralism in both buying and selling affects the behaviour of both providers and purchasers. Otherwise, providers rely on local income or purchasers can 'screw down' local providers.

Dependence on the local HA depends on the type of trust with a significantly smaller reliance by acute trusts on their local HA ($p < 0.001$). They had a median of 68% of income from host HAs compared to 78% for community and 76% for combined trusts. Acute trusts tended to get more from other HAs (10%). However, despite an apparent decline in the relative proportion of income derived from the local HA over time, there remains a heavy dependence by providers upon their host HA.

Figure 4.3 shows the breakdown of sources of average provider incomes from the second survey.

Seventy percent of trusts reported that they thought income from local HAs would reduce over time while the proportion of income obtained from GPFHs would gradually increase. Trusts were divided in opinion as to the prospective impact of non-local purchasers. Of our sample, 38 thought income from these would increase, 36 said it would decrease and the rest believed there would be no change. It is apparent that a slight overall shift is evident when considering the 'market' and current sources of income, although the picture is complicated and will be influenced by a variety of local factors. For example, in considering the range for the three major sources of income, we can observe considerable differences between provider units: local HA income ranges from 2% to 96% of a trust's income, other HAs less than 1% to 98%; GPFHs less than 1% to 60%. While one cannot conclude at a glance the character of the exceptions, a presumption might be that the locality of the provider, the

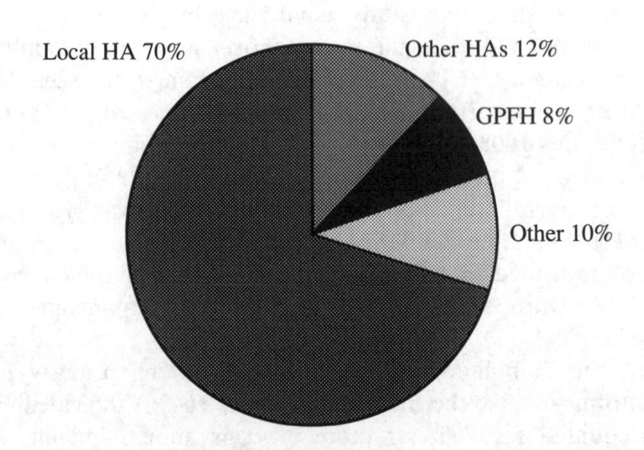

Figure 4.3. Breakdown of source of average provider income (based on means)

salience of GP fundholding and the type of provider unit will play a dominant part in dictating a provider's source of income.

Thus, one would obviously anticipate that a provider who is on the border between two HA areas is less likely to be dependent upon a single HA for income than a provider in the centre of a district. Likewise, the proximity of provider units within areas is also likely to influence income (i.e. if the unit is one of several within a relatively small geographical area). Similarly, the presence (or absence) of total fundholding practices, standard GPFHs and GPFH consortia will affect the local situation with regard to potential purchasers. In respect of the characteristics of the provider unit, the services which are provided may themselves determine the range of purchasers. For example, the response from a single specialty hospital indicated that their major sources of income was not their host HA (host HA 7%; other HAs 49%; GPFH 15%; other 29%).

While the tendency for providers to rely upon a single source of income may have implications for the purchaser/provider relationship, this can only be regarded as one aspect of the picture. An equally salient factor is the extent to which a single provider makes up a significant proportion of a purchaser's budget, i.e. is there symmetry in dependency?

The results from the first phase of the study highlighted that, just as providers are, by and large, heavily dependent upon a single income source, so HAs are dependent on a single provider (although not to the same degree). The typical HA was likely to allocate about half of its budget (median figure) to its main provider and, in the majority of cases, at least 70% of an HA's budget went to just three providers and at least 80% to just five providers. Only 20% tended to be allocated to providers outside their boundary. The primary reason for this is probably the result of an HA's resident population requiring the majority of its health care within easy access.

The larger percentages allocated outside boundaries tended to be in large urban areas such as London and Birmingham. Numbers of providers tended to range from 11 to 91 although this tended to be correlated with the size of an HA's budget.

While around half the trusts seemed confident that 'market forces' would come into play with more of their income being derived from outside their local HA, HAs themselves believed more in the locality of providers with 23 of the 37 HAs who answered the question in the first stage of the project believing less would be allocated to providers outside their boundaries in the future and only six thinking there would be an increase (the rest said no change). Of these six, five currently allocated less than the average for the respondent HAs outside their boundaries. It thus appears that HAs do not believe that greater market competition will come into force where HAs cross boundaries more often to obtain services. If HAs are increasingly to drive developments, this may be salient.

INTERPRETING THE RESULTS SO FAR

Data reported above, alongside follow-up in case studies, suggest that the contracting system, post-reform, has tended to replicate pre-reform arrangements. Whether or not purchasers and providers deal with single providers and purchasers (or a diversity) is less to do with the operation of a market and its facilitation of new decisions than old variations. Some of these are commonplace. A rural health authority may deal with one hospital. A health authority equidistant between four urban hospitals, on the other hand, will contract with more providers. This is not the same as 'potential for competition', however – it may merely reflect desired referral patterns specialty by specialty and clinical decisions overall. To explore more fully the scope for competition, one would have to compare homogeneous specialties in defined degrees of proximity to each other and then investigate the actual prospects for switching referrals (see Appleby *et al.*, 1994).

Where contracts have changed significantly, it has usually been as a result of mergers between hospitals; closures of specialties within providers (or of whole hospitals); or new services. Such changes are planned and managed by regions (now regional offices of the NHS executive), as individual trusts need to be 'managed from above' to produce such change. Indeed, the autonomy given to units within previously integrated health authorities makes the management of change more difficult.

The implications of all this for the purchaser/provider relationship is that HAs are liable to have a significant influence upon the activities and decisions of their local providers. Provider influence over the dominant purchaser is likely to be less significant, since the HA is not equally dependent upon them as a source of provision. However, it is possible that the provider influence, even in the typical situation, may be fairly strong. For example, a provider which is centrally located within a health district may have a significant influence over the local HA if the large majority of the provider's patients are all from a fixed catchment area with no alternative source of health care provision, i.e. there is a local monopoly. Similarly, as in the case of designated regional or national centres, the specificity of the service (as opposed to the location) may mean that the hospitals are able to influence purchasers to a greater degree given their niche in the marketplace (what would formerly have appeared as their planned pre-eminence).

Indeed, contracting for regional or national specialised services after the reforms has often been highly problematic. Instead of national or regional top-slicing (which still exists, but to a much lesser extent), which earmarks money for the services, local purchasers have to agree to joint contracts to ensure adequate finance for the service. This can be done by regional co-ordination of purchaser agreement by the purchasers themselves or at provider instigation, leading to political resolution. All these methods are roundabout. The advantage of devolving purchasing even for specialised, supra-health authority services is allegedly that individual purchasers can then fund more precisely what they need. This assumes that they know, of course; it might be a question of predicting in advance how many major heart operations there will be in the district over the next year or more.

Additionally, even when services are desired, there may be a 'problem of collective action' whereby each purchaser (logically) thinks there is only a point in contracting if others do the same. It is rather like paying tax – even if one assumes altruism and willingness to pay in principle, there is no point in paying unless the 'critical mass' of tax collected is enough for the purpose. What we have here is the difficulty in mobilising co-operative action even when it is desired by the individual actors.

Indeed, this could be a paradigm of the reforms: they have devolved decision making to inappropriate levels for certain types of service and 'recovering the situation' ironically is time consuming and bureaucratic.

CONTRACTING: STAFFING AND MARKETING

The number of staff in health authorities actually involved in assessing providers varied between one whole time equivalent (WTE) and 30 WTE. This is closely related to size of budget and overall numbers of staff ($p < 0.001$) and appears to have no relationship to the factors considered important by HAs in setting contracts. So, it does not seem to be the case from this limited analysis that HAs spend less time assessing providers if they consider location and current tenure of a contract as most important.

This point about provider power is reinforced by looking at what HAs considered most important in setting contracts. Cost and quality both had supporters but the same number of HAs placed location and (a similar number again) providers currently holding a contract as most important. Volume only became popular as a second priority.

Location becomes an important factor since it will represent an additional cost to patients and their friends or relatives if travelling is required to a hospital distant from their home. Thus, quite simply, it appears local providers dominate HA purchasing since the combined product that they supply is less costly than their non-local rivals and the reason for this domination is that currently there is insufficient difference between providers with regard to other aspects of the health-care product to outweigh the travelling costs connected to location.

However, the fact that almost half of the HAs were most concerned about location (and who currently held the contract) suggests that the NHS market is a limited affair and that geographical advantages (and having a foot in the door already) are just as important, if not more so, as cost, quality and volume which are treated as of secondary importance by most HAs. Some HAs have different views on the most important factors, with location considered as only the fourth most important factor by one in four HAs, but this is not the mainstream picture.

While a principal objective of the 1989 NHS reforms was to create a competitive market in the provision of health-care services via the separation of purchasers and providers, the relative importance of local influences remains strong, as we have seen. This is borne out by the comparatively low priority that trusts have given to developing the marketing function within their unit. If one considers that within a free market the need to 'sell' services is of major importance, it is apparent that most trusts do not regard this strategic objective as of particular significance. That is to say, while three-quarters of trusts indicated that there was an explicit responsibility for marketing at senior management level, the whole time equivalent dedicated to this function was typically less than one. Of those trusts with a specific senior management responsibility for purchasing, only 23% indicated that one senior management WTE was dedicated to marketing and a further 20% responded that they had more than one senior manager WTE with a specific marketing role.

Only one-quarter of trusts indicated that they had a marketing department within their unit (although this varied between acute trusts at 37%, combined at 32% and community trusts at 19%), with 55% of these having staff consisting of less than two WTE. Twenty-three percent indicated they had neither a marketing department nor senior management responsibility for marketing as, obviously, it is important to target actual function rather than title. Although, therefore, responsibility for marketing is given a specific standing within many units, the overall salience attached to this function in typical provider units may be regarded as relatively minor. Despite the purchaser/provider split, therefore, the perceived need to develop an internal marketing function as a means to attract income would seem to vary considerably.

Explanation of results

The need to market services depends crucially upon the degree of threat to those services. In a contracting market (the hospital sector in the NHS, for example) threat is more salient than opportunity. Where 'attack is the best form of defence', of course, the two may be intertwined: a trust may seek to persuade purchasers or regional or national planners that it is best to offer (for example) the oncology service, or whatever, to prevent it losing its reputation as an innovator, which may have 'knock-on' negative effects.

Where services are stable and 'monopolistic' (or, if market language is inappropriate, simply the local service!), marketing may be a waste of money for both provider and purchaser.

Also, some trusts and not others will be heavily into marketing to the extent that their managers are captivated by playing market games. This may not always bear much relation to objective needs or realities.

What sort of marketing?

In the second questionnaire, respondents were also asked to comment on the degree to which marketing was performed centrally rather than by specialty. This is an important decision for trust boards, as a common complaint from senior clinicians, including clinical directors (the managerial heads of their departments), is that they are bound by marketing decisions and contractual negotiations between purchaser and provider but not party to them. Thirty-eight percent of trusts indicated that any marketing within the unit tended to be mainly undertaken on a central basis, 17% performed mainly by the specialty and 45% equally. This is highlighted in Figure 4.4. There was little difference between the types of trust.

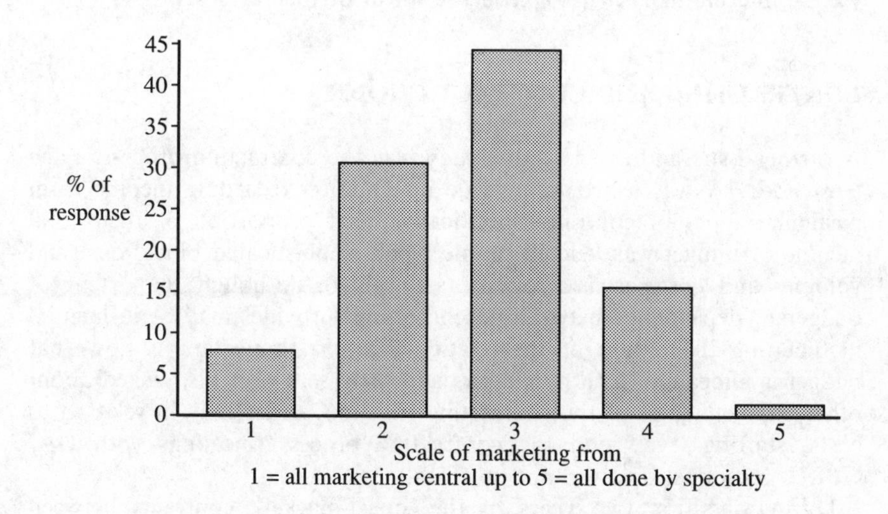

Figure 4.4. Where marketing is performed within trusts, on a scale of 1–5.

Again, it could be argued that this orientation results from a number of local circumstances. One single specialty hospital, for example, with a heavy reliance on income from sources other than the local HA, indicated that they had a department within the hospital specifically dedicated to marketing, three WTE senior marketing managers and an annual marketing budget of £100 000. While staff and associated departmental running costs obviously have impact on the costs of the marketing function, the degree to which trusts market their services is highlighted by the diversity of costs associated with marketing *per se*; 31 trusts provided details of their annual marketing budget, with such costs ranging from £2000 to £454 000. The median budget for a marketing department was £60 000. The median amount spent on the department for community trusts was 0.16% of income (interquartile range (IQR) 0.11%, 0.31%). Acute trusts spent 0.11% (IQR 0.04%, 0.18%) and combined trusts spent a median of 0.18% (IQR 0.04%, 0.30%).

It is not surprising, therefore, to find that comments relating to the marketing function varied considerably between trusts. Marketing was described by some trusts as having a 'low emphasis' or being 'limited' while other trusts highlighted the central advisory function of senior management (i.e. 'central expertise' available, 'expertise on costs', 'advisory function'). Other units adopted a different approach, saying that 'all staff are marketeers' and a minority of respondents indicated that there was specific responsibility for marketing services within specialties. Whether marketing is centrally or departmentally done, positions such as 'marketing manager' tend to be peripheral. The 'key players' do it and yet the internal market has spawned a lot of peripheral posts.

CONTRACTING AND CONTRACT CHOICE

A further issue addressed in the study was the contracting process. Each trust and HA was asked to provide information regarding income from particular types of contract: specifically, what proportion of their total income or budget was held in simple block; sophisticated block; cost and volume; and cost-per-case format (see below). Although the extent of budgetary dependency between purchaser and provider may be influential in dictating the nature of the relationship, also important is how that budget is allocated. Both purchasers and providers were also asked about other characteristics of the contracting function, specifically in relation to costs, staffing levels and the contracting process (meetings with HA/GPFH, personnel involved and so forth.).

During the first two years of the 'quasi-market', contracts between purchasers and providers varied considerably, primarily as a result of differing local circumstances. Despite such variation, however, three major types of contract were evident: block contracts, cost and volume contracts and cost-per-case contracts.

Originally, with a dearth of information, contracts in the internal market were designed to be of a generic nature (not case or event specific). Under such arrangements, patient access to a defined range of services and facilities is provided in return for a fixed annual fee. Such 'block' contracts were seen at the time as a temporary arrangement and in the longer term, as information sources and flows improved, it was envisaged that there would be a move towards more specificity within contracts (Appleby *et al.*, 1994). Therefore, one might anticipate that, at least five years on from the reforms, the majority of contracts will be of a more specific nature and block contracts will be in decline.

For the purposes of equity amongst respondents, a definition of sophisticated block was provided in the questionnaire which accorded with the NHSE Purchasing Unit's definition of the key contracting types.

- *Simple block:* purchasers pay the provider a fixed sum for access to a defined range of services or facilities. Such contracts may include some form of indicative workload agreement or fixed volume.
- *Sophisticated block:* purchasers pay providers a fixed contract sum for access to a defined range of services or facilities. Indicative patient activity targets or thresholds with 'floors' and 'ceilings' are included in such contracts, as well as agreed mechanisms if targets are exceeded. Elements of case mix may be included.
- *Cost and volume:* this type of contract specifies outputs in terms of patient treatment rather than inputs in terms of services or facilities available. Purchasers do not necessarily purchase fixed volumes, but will sometimes develop contracts with a fixed price being paid up to a certain volume of treatment and a price per case being paid above it, up to a volume ceiling.
- *Cost per case:* the hospital agrees to provide a range of specified treatments in line with a given contract price for individual cases.

When one examines the nature of contracts between providers and HAs it is evident that simple block and sophisticated block contracts account for the majority. Whether the nature of the contract type is a result of purchaser or provider preference is, however, a moot point, and one which will be dealt with in a later section.

As Figure 4.5 illustrates, almost one-quarter of providers indicated that 100% of their HA income was held in simple block contracts and a further 36.5% indicated that the entirety of their HA income was held in sophisticated block format. The remainder of trusts reported that income from HAs was obtained through a variety of differing contract types.

Trusts were also asked to provide details of the breakdown of their GPFH income as they did for HAs. While the earlier analysis highlighted

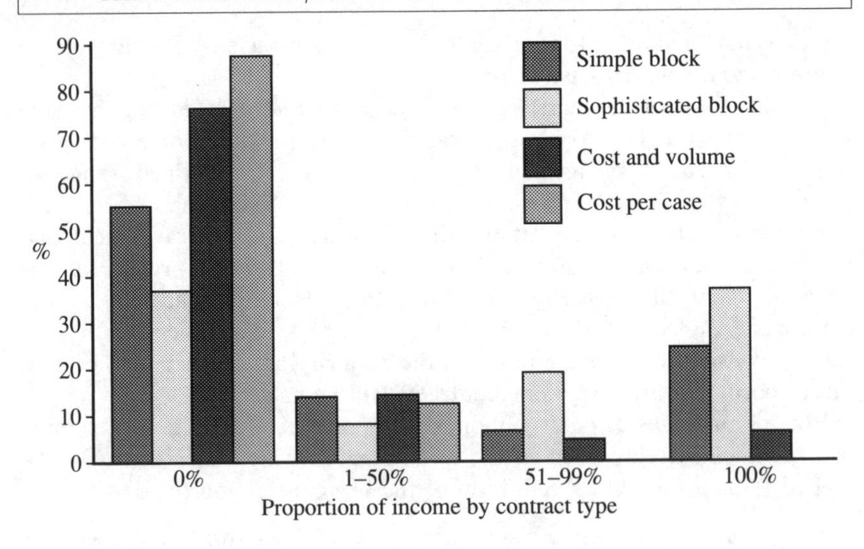

Figure 4.5. Major type of contract held between HAs and provider units.

that contracts between trusts and HA purchasers were predominantly held in some form of block contract, the type of contract established between trusts and GPFH showed a much high degree of variation, as illustrated in Figure 4.6). Such differentiation between purchaser groups and contract types is perhaps reflective of the number of episodes of care that each purchaser is procuring and the degree to which purchasers or providers are able to influence the nature of contracts themselves. Cost-per-case contracts, for example, are defined at the level of individual patient episodes and involve a considerable level of transactions costs. Accordingly, from both a purchaser and provider perspective, such formats are not conducive to high levels of contract activity, but may therefore be more suited to GPFHs.

Explanation of results

The predominance of the block format as the favoured type of contract in the second phase of the study highlights that comparatively little progress has been made in the move towards more cost-specific purchasing. Is this a matter of time or a deliberate strategy on the part of either managers or politicians? Block contracts have advantages for purchasers, in terms of 'buck passing', and (to a lesser extent) for providers in terms of simplicity (Paton, 1995).

The extensive use of more specific contracts by GPFHs could be a result of the GPFHs' marginal nature at the time of the survey. If fund-

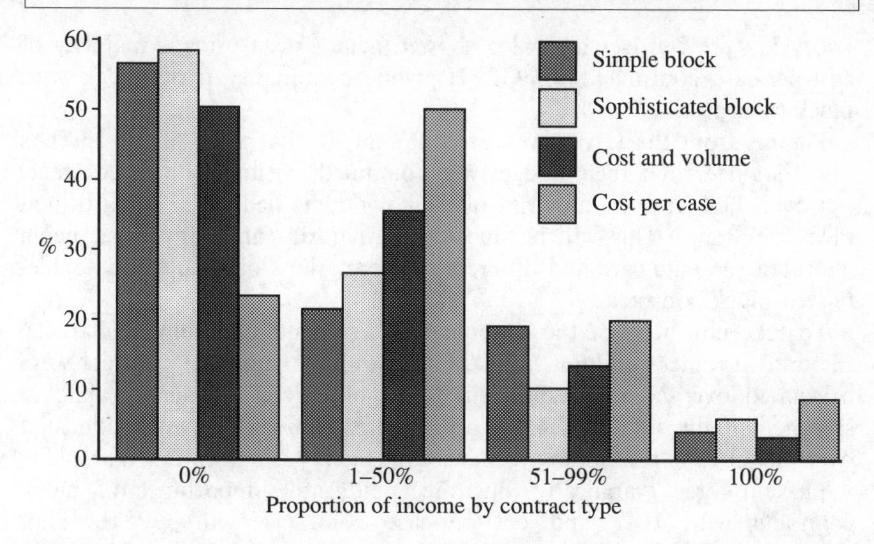

Figure 4.6. Major type of contract held between GPFHs and provider units.

holding becomes the norm, then reducing intolerable transactions costs might actually force their contracts into cost per volume or even block, as consortia of fundholders become the 'new health authorities'.

While the transactions costs per unit of running a cost-per-case contract are unlikely to be less for a GPFH than for an HA, if the GPFH is dealing in smaller total sums the extent of such costs may prove more acceptable. As the total sums increase, this will change. As more GPFH practices become multifunds, GPFH consortia or total purchasing sites, however, a trend for GPFH contracts to be held in cost and volume or even block formats may be established.

There was, however, discrepancy between types of contract and type of trust. Only 10% of acute trusts had the majority (greater than 50%) of HA income in the form of simple block contracts as opposed to 35% of combined trusts and 42% of community trusts. Sixty-eight percent of acute trusts, however, had the majority of their HA income in the form of sophisticated block, as opposed to 50% of community and 48% of combined trusts.

The major difference came in the form of contracts with GPFHs ($p < 0.001$). Only one acute trust had the majority of their GPFH income in the form of a simple block contract but 40% of community trusts and two of the 23 combined trusts had the simple block contract dominant. Acute trusts were much more likely to use a majority of cost-per-case contracts with GPFHs (55%) compared to just 5% of community and 43% of combined trusts. This result was very similar to the first survey two years previously which also showed acute trusts using a majority of cost-per-case contracts with GPFHs while community trusts stuck with block contracts.

Figures from the HA survey are different, in that none of the 33 HAs said that over half their budget was contained in simple block contracts but over 70% had the majority of their contracts tied up in sophisticated block contracts. This will be due to the majority of their budget being allocated to acute care and different interpretations of simple and sophisticated block contracts.

To take into account the larger incomes of acute and combined trusts, the total incomes resulting from the four different types of contract were calculated over all the respondent trusts of the second survey and are shown in Figures 4.7 and 4.8. Furthermore, how the budget is allocated over the 33 HAs responding to the second survey is shown in Figure 4.9.

These figures graphically illustrate, firstly, the importance of block contracts with HAs and cost-per-case contracts with GPFHs and, secondly, the much higher incomes of acute and combined trusts.

PREFERRED CONTRACTS AND ACTUAL CONTRACTS

That the provider units may be unable to determine the format of local contracts is highlighted by the disparity which exists between actual and

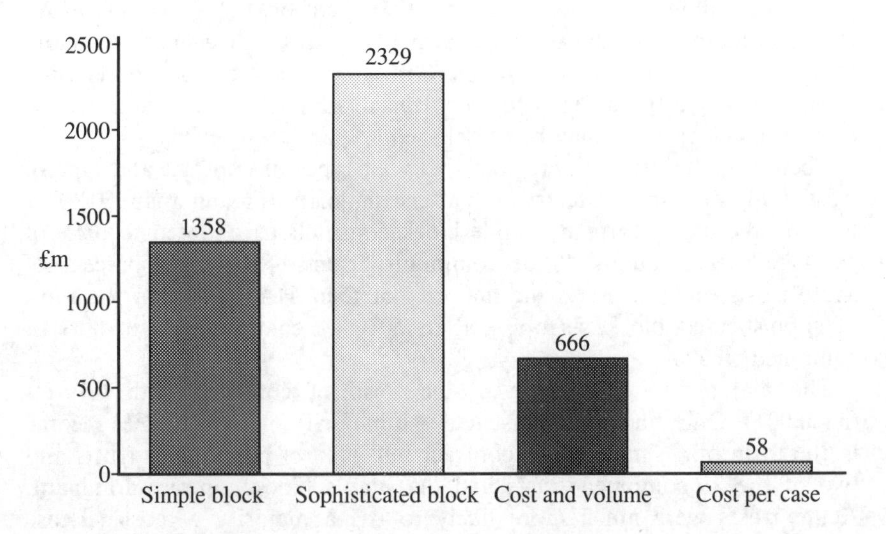

Figure 4.7. Total income generated by contract type with HAs over all respondent trusts.

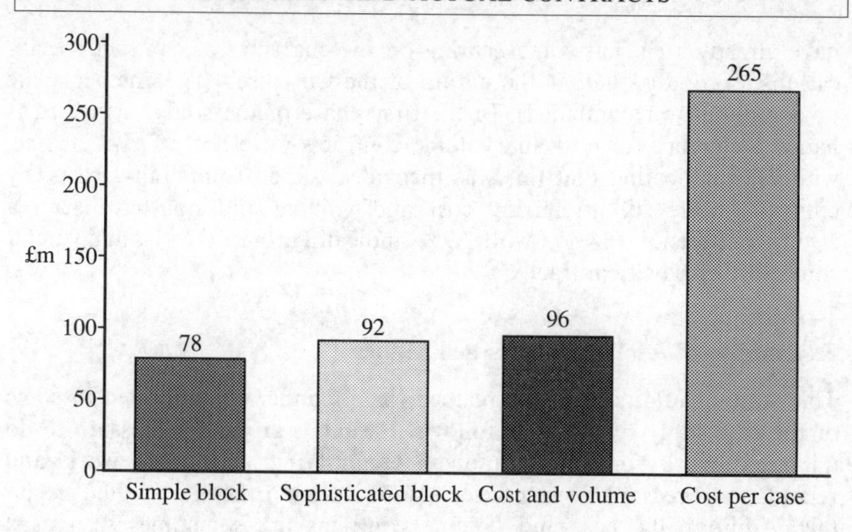

Figure 4.8. Total income generated by contract type with GPFHs over all respondent trusts.

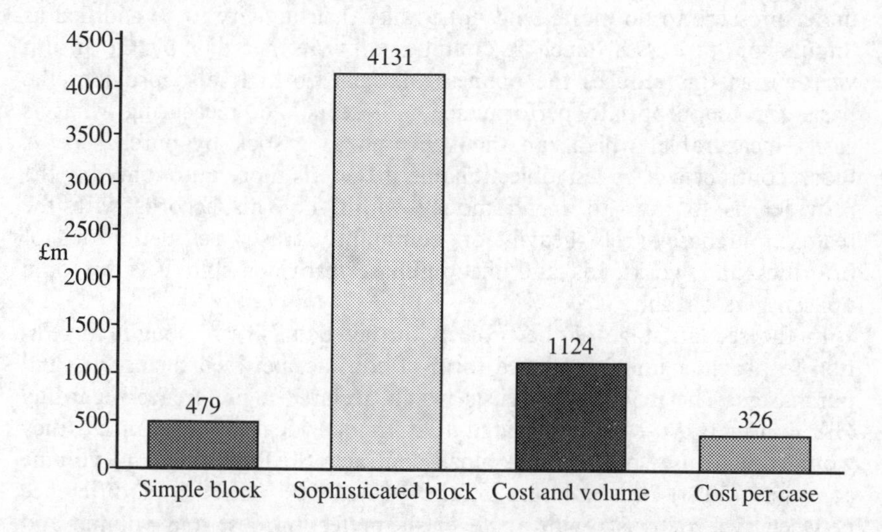

Figure 4.9. Budget allocation of HAs by contract type over all respondents.

preferred types of contract held. All groups participating in the study were asked about which contract format they would prefer (if not that currently held) and the reasons for any disparity. Trusts could be separated in their replies on two counts.

Firstly, there is the nature of the purchaser (HA/GPFH), which, as we have already seen, has some bearing on the character of contract specifications. Secondly, there is the nature of the trust itself (i.e. whether acute or community or combined). In the first phase of the study, acute trusts had a preference for cost and volume contracts in respect of HA income, with 77% indicating that this was their ideal state. Community trusts, by contrast, while still preferring cost and volume, did not have such a strong preference (54%), with 39% indicating that they would prefer some sort of block contract.

Explanation of results: analytics and politics

This state of affairs can be explained (in a manner corroborated in some of the case study research) as follows. Hospitals are under pressure to do unlimited work for limited money. Quantifying reasonable work and relating it to reasonable income (cost and volume) therefore suited hospitals. Additionally, cost and volume contracts are sometimes seen as a middle way and therefore a compromise which allows agreement between purchaser and provider. Community units, on the other hand, while still under pressure to do more, tend not to like their activity to be codified as 'inputs' or 'processes' (such as 'number of visits per day by the health visitor'), as this reduces the richness of their work. It also provides the basis for inappropriate performance indicators, i.e. measuring what is easily measurable, which can then be used as a stick by purchasers. A block contract will be less objectionable if there is more autonomy for the provider as to how to spend money within it. This accords with the reality: purchasers rely heavily on community trusts' self-definitions of priorities and workloads and the purchaser/provider split is a bit of a nonsense as a result.

In the second stage of the project, further details were sought in relation to provider units' preferred form of contract between themselves and purchasers. The majority of trusts which declared a preference regarding HA contracts ($n = 110$) indicated that, under ideal circumstances, they would opt to use sophisticated block contracts (41.8%), cost and volume contracts (30%) or a mixture of the two (18%). There is a difference between type of trust, with acute trusts preferring cost and volume and sophisticated block contracts equally and community trusts preferring sophisticated block. Only a small minority of trusts highlighted a preference for cost-per-case (6.3%) contracts.

Differences between the surveys could be interpreted perhaps as trusts not wanting simple block contracts but something more activity based (there was no separation of simple and sophisticated block contracts in the first survey). Otherwise trusts can be 'squeezed' – fixed money but variable (i.e. increasing) workload. The 'efficiency savings' of 3% sought annually by the government and the rule that price must equal cost may indeed make the difference between types of contract rather academic: there is prescribed or necessary workload and limited income!

When considering the nature of contracts held with GPFHs, those trusts expressing a preference ($n = 120$) rated sophisticated block contracts and cost and volume contracts equally (25.8%). In contrast to contracts held with HA purchasers, some trusts highlighted that cost-per-case contracts and a mix of cost and volume/cost-per-case contracts were also desirable when contracting with GPFHs.

In the first stage of the project, 22 of the 28 HAs who expressed a preference for one type of contract named cost and volume contracts, while the remaining six named block contracts. Nobody went solely for cost-per-case, possibly as the costs of operating such specific contracts are too excessive. The second stage gave differing results with seven of the 33 HAs preferring cost and volume, 15 preferring sophisticated block and six preferring a combination of the two. There seem to be differences within HAs as to their preferred type of contract and, possibly, a confusion over the difference between sophisticated block contracts and cost and volume (even though these were defined on the questionnaire in the second stage). Again, though, there is a desire to move away from simple block contracts.

While the above yields some interesting results, it does not explain why particular contracting patterns are occurring between different purchaser and provider combinations. Indeed, it adds further complications to the questions for which answers are being sought. Given the preference for sophisticated block contracts or cost and volume contracts under many of the scenarios, why is there still a widespread use of simple block contracts? For example, almost one in four trusts indicated that 100% of HA contracts were held in simple block format yet no trust indicated a preference for this type of contract.

Wider political realities, again – in opposition to the rhetoric of more sophisticated contracting – may contain the explanation. As the costs of a sophisticated market become known, both in terms of running it and in terms of revealing ‘underfunding’, the government may put other imperatives above the fully ‘costed out’ (let alone market-driven) NHS.

RELATIONSHIPS WITHIN CONTRACTS

In addition to asking HAs and trusts what their contract preferences were, respondents were also asked to indicate the reason for that preference, which can give an indication of how particular types of contracts are being used in particular relationships and who (the purchaser or provider) is dominating the relationship.

The first stage of the project revealed that in the case of providers (both acute and community), the dominant reason for wanting more activity-based contract types when contracting with HAs was that under such contracts income would better reflect activity. Other reasons regarded as significant were guaranteed income and reduced risk. It would appear, therefore, that the reason why providers wish to move away from simple block contracts and into more specific contracts is that currently the money that they receive for the services they supply is not necessarily assured. In a perfect market, the response of the provider/supplier would be not to supply services other than those they have been contracted for, even if this was in disagreement with the purchaser, since it would imply that their costs would be greater than their revenue and they would go out of business.

Since the implication is that purchasers can gain additional activity at no extra cost under the terms of a simple block contract, it would appear that some of the conditions of a perfect market are not in operation and purchasers have a 'bargaining advantage' over providers. Despite the preferences given in the first stage of the study as to contract type and the stated objective on the part of provider units of wishing to reduce risk and secure income, the comparatively low use of cost and volume and cost-per-case contracts suggests that trusts are unable to influence contract negotiations as much as they would wish. Alternatively, given the generally high level of activity purchased by HAs, the practicalities of using cost and volume or cost-per-case contracts render such contract types unmanageable for the large volume of HA work.

This is suggested by trusts, as when asked why contracts had not been changed to the type the trust preferred (if different to current type), the two most common answers were that it was due to the unwillingness of HAs to change, coupled with poor information systems making cost and volume contracts difficult.

As the NAHAT (1994) highlights, however, in examining the reasons why particular purchasers and providers have adopted a certain format of contract, to focus largely on the concept of 'risk' may ignore other determining factors. Additionally, in many purchaser/provider relationships, to make a clear distinction regarding risk (i.e. to whom and under what circumstances is the risk higher?) is artificial in that often the provider's risk is also the purchaser's risk, especially in situations where a monopoly exists (a single trust being the major provider for a local HA, with no realistic alternatives). This may partly explain why no HA preferred a simple block contract in the second survey.

The first phase of the study explored both purchaser and provider perceptions of who took the lead in the contract specification process and a significant difference was apparent between acute and community trust responses regarding this issue ($p < 0.05$). Community trusts were more likely to say that they led (18 out of 34 responses) rather than the purchaser (5/34). Acute trusts, by contrast, said that they led (13/36) compared to 14/36 where the purchaser led. The remainder of the responses indicated that the lead in the contracting process was split 50:50. While such results may arise as a result of the nature of the contract or local circumstances or may reflect a bias in the response, they nonetheless highlight that the relationship between purchasers and providers is variable. These results, nevertheless, differ from how HAs see the contracting process; thirteen (37%) HAs said they led the contracting process and only four said it was the provider that led. Eighteen said it was 50:50. The difference between the acute trusts' version of events and HAs', significant for the respondents ($p < 0.01$), seems to be in the definition of the HA defined '50:50' contracts, with providers seeming to believe they normally lead these.

Similar discrepancies exist in the specifying of contracts between GPFHs and trusts. GPFHs said input to a contract's specification was either mainly through them (20 respondents) or 50:50 with the provider (21 respondents). Only six said that the trust led the process. Once more, there was disagreement as to who had the most input in a contract's specification; 37 of the 70 trusts who responded said they had the greatest input compared to only 15 who said it was the GPFHs (the rest stated it was 50:50).

The importance of purchaser input into the contracting process is that, without it, the purchaser is open to exploitation by the provider – the provider can develop a contract that is in its interest, rather than the general interest of the purchaser (and, by implication, the public or patient). Effectively, the supplier is acting as an agent to the purchaser (though the purchaser may not be aware of it) and may operate in an imperfect manner to maximise its own 'utility function' rather than that of the purchaser. Both trusts and HAs can supply expertise to the process, but it is the provider which supplies the substantive knowledge while the purchaser is devoting its efforts to conducting the process and arriving at formal contracts.

It may be that HAs are more knowledgeable about acute services than community services and, therefore, necessarily need a greater input from community trusts than acute trusts. Regardless of how the two sides are brought together, what we are observing (if the providers are believed) is that there exists a greater asymmetry in information between purchasers and providers in community care than there is in acute care. Hence one might expect to observe a greater use of block contracts by purchasers so as to overcome this knowledge disadvantage. This, however, leaves purchasers open to manipulation either when there is low demand for services or in the manner in which a service is provided.

Here, the 'purchaser/provider split' may reduce effectiveness of service stipulation and delivery, as co-operation is replaced by 'gaming' and the perverse initiatives of an (inevitably) imperfect market come into play.

THE ORGANISATION OF CONTRACTING

Despite the rapid development of contracting over the past few years, highlighted by the increase in the average number of contracts from 16 to 30 for a typical provider (NAHAT, 1994), only 43% of trusts in the current study indicated that they had a department solely concerned with contracting (no difference between type of trust). Only one in three HAs had a department concerned solely with contracting, with budgets ranging between £60 000 and £470 000 (median £174 000). There tended to be between five and 15 WTE HA personnel with specific contracting roles (median 8).

The expansion of contracting in relation to purchaser numbers (primarily as a result of the growth in GPFHs) has implications for the contract workload in terms of negotiations, documentation, administration and possible workload variation in patient activity. This in turn results in an additional category of expenditure that was not incurred under the pre-reform unitary system. As has been illustrated, the majority of trusts have either developed a specific department for contracting or have a number of personnel dedicated to contract management.

Further costs arising from the introduction of the internal market can be seen when considering the establishment and monitoring of contracts. In relation to the number of meetings typically required between purchasers and providers to set up a contract, not only was there great variation but differences were also apparent according to types of purchaser. Eighty-six percent of trusts normally had between one and three meetings with a GPFH but only 24% had similar numbers with HAs. The majority of trusts had between three and ten meetings with HAs; this was confirmed by figures from the HA survey.

The typical length of these meetings, for 80% of respondents, was between two and three hours for provider/HA meetings and between one and two hours for contract meetings between providers and GPFH purchasers. The response from HAs was only slightly different, with 75% saying typical meetings lasted between 1.5 and three hours. This, of course, has ramifications when trusts are providing services to a large number of purchaser groups. With GP fundholding increasing rapidly in many areas, a large amount of time will be taken up with GPFHs who make up a disproportionate amount of time in contract meetings for providers in relation to the size of their contract.

Table 4.1. Number of meetings held between trusts and providers in order to establish contract.

No. of meetings	*HA- % of providers*	*GPFH- % of providers*
1-2	9.6	60.1
3-4	34.9	30.5
5-6	19.9	5.1
7-8	8.9	0.7
9-10	7.5	–
11-12	11.0	0.7
13+	8.2	2.9

Invariably, the number of people from trusts who attended contract meetings with GPFHs was less than HAs. The increasing number of GPFHs and their relative importance in terms of income were likely to dictate this. The only difference between types of trust was that acute trusts tended to have only one member from specialties at meetings with HAs. There was agreement between trusts and HAs as to the median number of people who took part in contract meetings.

Table 4.2. Median number of personnel involved at contract meetings.

Personnel from	*HA meetings*	*GPFH meetings*
Central trust	3	2
Specialty	2	1
Purchaser	4	2

As has already become clear, the establishment of the purchaser/provider split and the development of contracting has resulted in substantial costs. While many of the costs associated with such change (i.e. setting up systems for costing of services, patient information systems, billing, recording and monitoring) are non-recurring, other costs will persist as a result of the continuing transactions between purchasers and providers.

CONTRACT NEGOTIATIONS

Under perfect market conditions, the principal factor which provides purchasers with an indication as to the products or services which they buy is cost. Few markets are perfect however, and the 'internal' and 'quasi' market within the NHS, while demonstrating some principles of the marketplace (in, for example, the separation of purchasing from provision, some competition and the development of contracting), is also managed and regulated in a variety of ways. That is to say, contracts may be placed with provider units for a variety of reasons and purchasers' contractual intentions may be influenced by a variety of not necessarily compatible concerns.

From a provider perspective, however (and despite the emphasis placed on the quality of service provision within contracts), the overwhelming majority of provider units felt that, when it came to negotiating contracts, HAs placed *cost* as their principal concern (124 trusts placed it as the top or joint top priority). Activity (volume) was second highest priority (40) and the quality of service provision third (4).

GPFHs, by contrast, were regarded by trusts as having a somewhat different approach from HAs to contracting. Not surprisingly, given the mechanics of fundholding and the rising financial concerns of many practices which have become fundholders, cost was still regarded by the majority of trusts as the major concern of GPFHs when establishing contracts with provider units (91 trusts placed it as the top or joint top priority). However, the emphasis given to quality by GPFHs was perceived by providers as much greater than HAs (33 trusts), as Figure 4.10 illustrates. The different types of trusts tended to have similar views on the priorities of

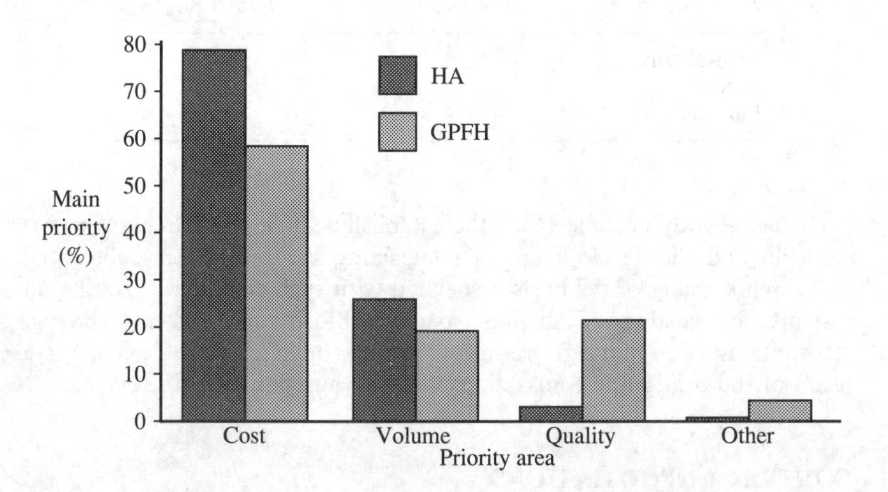

Figure 4.10. Perceived priorities of purchasers by trusts (NB: Total % is greater than 100 as some providers indicated that purchasers gave equal priority to more than one area).

their purchasers, although slightly more community trusts thought that GPFHs were more interested in volume than the other types. Trusts also thought that GPFHs were concerned about waiting times (the majority of the 'others') and direct referrals.

QUALITY

Almost half of the trusts stated that they rated quality as of much higher importance than they believed the HAs rated it. This is backed up by the previously mentioned results that quality was not, overall, deemed by HAs to be any more important than cost, location and the provider currently holding the contract when assessing providers for contracts. Furthermore, financial pressures are likely to leave providers frustrated as to quality, with health authorities more remote from the day-to-day implications as well as adjudicating between competing demands upon limited resources.

Such results may reflect the perceived advantages of GPFHs, as viewed from the perspective of the provider, in that they feel more able to determine the nature of their contracts (particularly quality specifications) as a result of the nature of the contract and activity purchased.

The priority perceived to be given to cost and volume by HAs in the current study contrasts with the findings of an earlier survey of HAs (NAHAT, 1994), which found that such purchasers reported that the quality of service provision was their primary concern and that failure in this area was a major factor influencing their decision to change contracts and/or contractors. Patient access to services and competitive prices were ranked second and third respectively, as was information on the cost effectiveness of treatments.

The changed result may reflect the samples, but may also indicate the growing 'squeeze'.

The evaluation of quality, however, would appear to be based on the role of the purchaser and its own concerns and priorities, as opposed to the quality of service provision as viewed by the users of such services. In the respective rankings of contractual performance (and factors which may determine change), for example, the views of local residents were rated as the least important element of contract performance/service quality.

PROVIDER ASPIRATIONS

Earlier, it was suggested that the agendas of purchasers and providers were not necessarily the same. To aid a greater appreciation of the purchaser/provider split and the determinants of service provision, trusts were also asked about their areas of 'strength' in the marketplace and those areas of service provision which they intended to develop over the next three years.

In the first phase of the study, providers were asked to indicate those services where they felt that they had a competitive advantage and what the nature of such an advantage was. Most trusts gave multiple answers – that is to say, a single distinct advantage was not usual – and a number of advantages were presented, depending upon the service concerned. Recording the frequency with which certain answers were given, the following can be observed: quality was stated as a competitive advantage by 73% of trusts, while monopoly status was indicated by 57%. Cost, although mentioned, was felt to be a competitive advantage in less than half of all cases (43%).

Respondents were also given the opportunity of highlighting any other advantage that they felt they possessed. These responses could broadly be categorised under two headings of reputation/advertising and location, where the latter was in many ways equivalent to monopoly status. The above, while informative as to the nature of the market, must be treated with caution since the questions only related to those areas of service provision where a distinct advantage was perceived to exist. Thus the results may not be an indication of what form competition is taking as a whole or to what extent technical efficiency can be said to be improving, since such services may be at the margin. In other words, it could be the case that for the majority of services competition is very intense and as a result, no single provider feels that it has a distinct advantage over other local providers.

If such results are taken at face value, the implication is that purchasers are frequently using criteria other than cost to select providers, and therefore the incentive for such providers to be technically efficient is not as great as it would be if purchasers were selecting a homogeneous product on cost or price alone.

PURCHASER ASPIRATIONS

One can examine these results in the context of earlier results from the NAHAT study which identified ease of travel for residents as a major concern for HAs (after quality and before competitive prices) in their purchasing strategy and also stressing the importance of both location and existing contracts from results of this study. It may well be that purchasers select sites for the purchase of services according to particular locally defined criteria but that once such a decision is made (and given the dependency relationship which tends to exist between local providers and purchasers) contract negotiation in the actual cost is then accorded a high level of significance.

Two-thirds of the respondent HAs from the first survey stated that they carried out 'joint purchasing' with other agencies or purchasers for certain types of care. These embraced a wide range of services but particularly mental health services, learning difficulties and community care. Commonly mentioned advantages of joint purchasing were greater purchasing power and sharing risk. However, only around 40% of trusts said they had contracts with joint purchasers.

MONITORING

With the rapid development of the purchaser/provider split and the introduction of contracting, HAs encountered a number of problems during the first few years following the reforms, the most notable of which was cited as a lack of good information (Le Grand, 1994). As alluded to earlier, the greater the specification of the contract, the higher will be the information requirement of that contract. As also highlighted previously, one of the principal reasons trusts did not change to more activity-based contracts related to poor information systems and the accuracy of data concerned with patient activity, GP referrals and the costing of services. Additional problems were apparent in relation to the monitoring of contracts, with the majority of HAs citing the lateness and poor quality of information from provider units as a major source of difficulty (NAHAT, 1994). Accordingly, the areas of contract monitoring and information formed a major component of the current study.

In the first stage of the current project, there was consensus between providers and HAs over the frequency of the monitoring of contracts by HAs to assess progress, monitor contracts and ensure that standards were being maintained. Approximately two-thirds of HAs indicated that they monitored contracts monthly and a large majority of the remaining HAs reported that monitoring of contracts was undertaken quarterly. Only a small minority monitored bi-monthly or semi-annually and there was no difference between types of trust.

Most trusts also indicated that they were in regular contact with local HAs in addition to the formal monitoring process, so there appears to be a continuing contact between purchasers and providers regarding contract activity throughout the financial year. However, to monitor effectively, the measurements of contract success or failure need to be effective and accurate and this leads on to the HA assessment of their contracts in general.

Almost three-quarters of HAs (stage 1) said that failure of providers to meet contract specifications had been a problem. Of these, meeting activity levels, meeting the Patient's Charter targets, quality and waiting times had been the major concerns. Concerns over activity levels mainly revolved around either underachievement or excess work for which payment was expected. The dominance of block contracts may explain the quantity failure as providers fail to deliver what was agreed and any incentive to hit contract targets is weakened as the budget will already have been allocated. Inadequate and late information was also cited as a concern for many HAs, although such problems are not new to the NHS. Patient's Charter and waiting list failures may be predictable as these are areas which are likely to be closely monitored, although one would anticipate that therefore there is every incentive for the provider to meet such targets.

Ironically, as previously stated, quality was mentioned by a number of trusts as an advantage for them over their competitors. This is, however, a relative concept: it is impossible to quantify whether such views related to moderate quality compared to poor quality or did indeed refer to high quality of services.

'OVERPROVISION'

In the second stage, HAs again believed that 'overprovision' (ten out of 33 placed it first), quality of information (7) and waiting list targets (6) were the main causes of failure in contracts. Overprovision means more health care provided than can be financially justified! It may be that some purchasers' contracts still have 'money left in the pot' whereas others do not. GP fundholders, for example, may still have money left to buy care, in the financial year, whereas the local health authority does not (unless it expects the provider to squeeze more out of the block contract). This assumes that no standard specialty or disease costing is used. The alternative – of national or regional specialty costs broken down into diagnosis-related costs – does not apply. As a result, providers can be squeezed. In Sweden, when diagnosis-related groups were used in certain counties to reimburse hospitals, provision rose and (in the absence of British-type block budgets) the only way to limit costs was to cut the reimbursement per case.

Quality, however, was not considered a main cause of failure of contracts. This may either be due to high quality provided by trusts or because trusts are correct in believing HAs are not so concerned about quality. Anecdotal evidence would strongly suggest the latter – whatever the ministerial rhetoric, purchasers know that they have to trade off quantity and quality.

Explanation

'Overprovision' is a post-reform concept, of course, in the sense that only contracted or 'expected' activity is legitimate! Targets for performance within trusts include limitations upon activity as well as incentives to greater activity. Money does not follow the patient and so 'overprovision' is a danger. The danger with innumerable contracts, each of which can lead to 'overprovision', is that there is less flexibility for planners and purchasers to ensure that overall needs among the population are either met or prioritised. The arbitrariness of access, depending upon who is one's purchaser and the financial state of the contract at time of medical need, is a major consequence of the reforms.

In those circumstances where contract activity exceeded agreed levels or there were other financial pressures within contracts, the majority of trusts (58.8%) indicated that there was an expectation on the part of the HA that it was up to the provider to sort out the situation (the primary reason being that the HA has no reserve finances to pay for extra activity). Although a further four out of ten providers reported that they worked with the local HA to try to manage the situation (possibly by looking at areas of underactivity and juggling the contract specifications), only 2% of trusts said that they received any extra money for additional work undertaken. This was the case across all the types of trust with over half being expected to sort it out by themselves. This result is contradicted by HAs where three-quarters said they would work with the provider to sort out financial pressures arising within contracts and only two of the 33 respondents said they would expect the provider to sort it out.

The second stage of the study highlighted that the monitoring of contracts was a major concern for all trusts, with six out of ten (60.9%) indicating that their main incentive for monitoring was in relation to assessing activity against finance. A further 20% of the sample reported that HA contract requirement monitoring was the second major incentive for monitoring! Self-knowledge was also an important reason for monitoring, with 55% placing it as either the main or second reason for monitoring. By contrast, national indicators and clinical audit, while rated by trusts as important, were ascribed less significance than a concern with contractual performance. This, perhaps, describes the importance of keeping purchasers happy and concentrating on the local area. Of course, if purchasers' targets reflect the need to obey national indicators, the circle is partly squared.

INFORMATION

In relation to information provision, the second phase of the study sought to establish the relative growth in the information function within trusts (although this does not necessarily reflect the quality of information that is produced, nor the development of systems to monitor contract activity accurately).

The median budget allocation for 1994–95 was £125 000 (IQR £80 000, £220 000). Acute trusts actually had smaller budgets allocated to information (median £100 000) compared to community (£140 000) and combined (£137 590) although the range for combined trusts was much wider, one combined trust reporting a budget of £1.5m compared to a maximum for community trusts of £580 000 and for acute of £752 000. The median was six WTE dedicated to this role in 1994–95; broken down by type, it was acute five, community six and combined six WTE.

The range (1–54.5), however, reflects the activity of the different trusts, existing structures and the development of information as a means to effecting the mechanics of the internal market on a local basis.

If one compares these figures for the periods 1990–91, 1992–93 and 1994–95, it is apparent that significant expansion of the information function within provider units has occurred. The differences between the different types of trusts remain throughout the time period as shown in Figures 4.11 and 4.12 (figures for 1990–91 should be treated with caution due to the lack of trusts able to give information for this financial year). Nevertheless, an interesting picture of 'pre- and post-reform' aims emerges.

Community trusts, in particular, have suffered the costs of information, especially, as our case studies showed, with poor information systems, lack of proper analysis, substantial demand, particularly from recent fundholders eager for every scrap of information, and lack of national guidelines on data which should be collected. Information has been a big cost issue for most trusts, often substantially more than the costs of marketing or contracting departments.

Costs of information departments in the two years between 1992–93

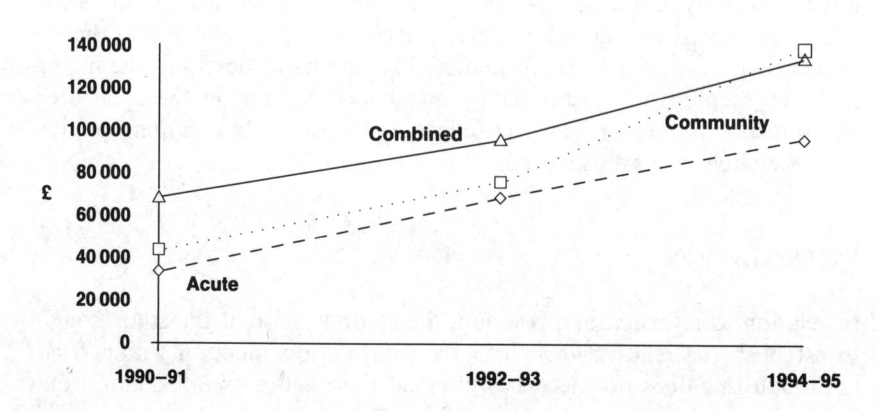

Figure 4.11. Median information department budget by type of trust.

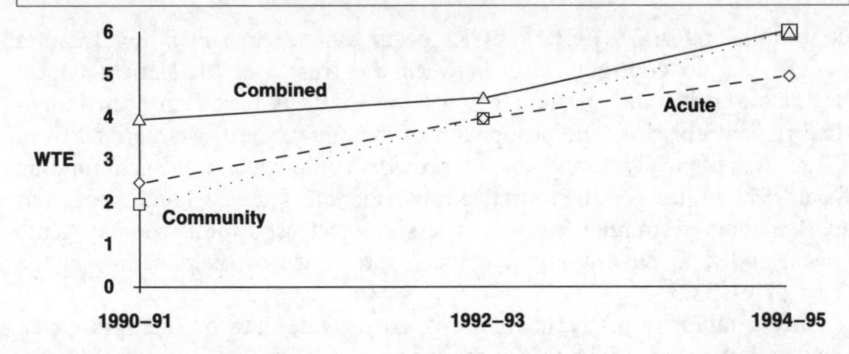

Figure 4.12. Median staff numbers in information department by type of trust.

Table 4.3. Information department budget/staffing over all trusts, 1990–95

	Median Budget	*Median WTE*
1990–91	£50 000	3
1992–93	£77 000	4
1994–95	£125 000	6

and 1994–95 have risen by a median 25% (IQR 4.5%, 58.8%) (£20 000) although 11 of the 64 trusts who gave information for both years had rises of more than 150%. Reflecting the lower starting point, acute trusts tended to have the biggest rise (33%) compared with community (25%) and combined (18%) although overall this difference is not statistically significant.

Information may be seen as a bolster to contracting and not a discrete activity, so the combined growth may be the most relevant figure. Legitimate needs for information, whose benefit outweighs its cost, are one thing. Most of the information requirements are however for short-term contracting and related requirements. This is the same issue as whether the NHS has too many managers. Investment in management is important, but investment in 'managers' to administer reams of data of dubious value, and use it in contracting, is wasteful.

EXTRACONTRACTUAL REFERRALS (ECRS) . . .

With the development of purchasing and the use of contracts to secure a wide range of services for local populations, we also examined extracontractual referrals (ECRs). ECRs occur when a provider unit treats a patient but no contract exists between the trust and the patient's local health authority and the unit of cost for ECRs is based on each individual patient episode. The proportion of income which trusts derived from ECRs was typically low: 95% of providers indicated that such funding forms 5% or less of their total annual income and 47% indicated that ECR income accounted for 1% or less of the trust's total income. Acute trusts tended to have a slightly higher percentage of their income in the form of ECRs.

Only a minority of trusts were able to provide data on changes which they had experienced in this area during the past three years, although where such information was provided, the figures ranged from a reduction of 50% to an increase of 500%. Such variation was accounted for by factors such as changing contracts (for example the failure of a contract which led to all cases from a particular HA being treated as ECRs during one specific financial year) or the establishment of contracts where none existed previously. Almost four out of ten providers, however, reported a static situation with regard to ECRs, the past three years having witnessed no change.

. . . AND EMERGENCIES

When looking at the proportion of ECRs which were classified as emergency treatment, it is apparent that the majority of ECRs fall into this category.

Six out of ten trusts which supplied data relating to this issue ($n=110$) indicated that emergency treatment formed more than half of all ECRs, with one in five trusts reporting that emergency ECRs formed 95–100% of their total ECR work. This would appear to be specific to local circumstances and/or the nature of the trust itself (i.e. the vast majority of ECR admissions to mental health trusts were cited as being emergencies). Combined trusts and community trusts tended to have a higher proportion of ECRs considered as emergencies (median of 90% and 70% respectively) compared to acute (60%, $p = 0.06$). Of the 28 trusts which supplied information on the changing pattern of emergency ECRs, the general tendency was no change over time, although again the range (–90% to +100%) was regarded by respondents as reflecting particular local events.

ECRs were not considered a large proportion of an HA's total budget, with no HA having more than 4% of their budget allocated for ECRs. However, when considered alongside the size of an HA's budget then it is a sizeable figure, around £2.5 million for an average HA. It was considered that around half the ECRs could be classified as emergency referrals by most HAs, although the figure rose to 80% for a couple of HAs.

The important question surrounding ECRs is the disproportionate cost and bureaucracy required to administer and service them. In effect, they represent the 'illegitimate' or unplanned episodes of care by the criteria of the reformed NHS, but necessary or desirable episodes by other criteria. Finding a better means of handling such referrals, which reimburses necessary care yet without bureaucracy and conflict on the present scale, is generally agreed to be necessary and was an area for action both under the previous Conservative government (under the aegis of the NHS efficiency unit) and under the Labour government after May 1997.

RELATIONSHIPS BETWEEN PROVIDERS

In the first survey the issue of relationships between acute and community trusts was addressed. Twenty-one trusts were unable to specify their relationship in terms of the three options on the questionnaire; 'complementary', 'competitive' and 'lead provider model'.

The 'lead provider' model is one in which, say, an acute trust subcontracts care for patients to a community trust or vice versa. The alternatives, to ensure continuous ('seamless') provision for patients requiring care in more than one location, are: for the purchaser to regulate or mandate inter-trust relations; for the trusts to behave co-operatively; or for a trust to take over (the other's) services. All in all, separate 'business-like' trusts may have rendered this process more difficult, with competitive forces and sharper financial imperatives leading to 'cost shifting' and 'patient dumping'.

Of the rest, there appeared a difference in working relationships between acute and community trusts. There was a significant difference between them with regard to the number of complementary and competitive relationships ($p < 0.05$) as detailed in Table 4.4.

Community trusts seem more likely to believe they have a competitive relationship with complementary services. This may be just a foible of the sample or due to different beliefs in the structure and working of the

Table 4.4. Relationships between complementary services

	Acute trusts	*Community trusts*	*Other trusts*
Complementary	20	12	8
Competitive	7	13	4
'Lead provider' Model	4	2	4
Other	7	6	8

relationship and/or how it should work. Half of the HAs in the survey said there were situations where providers appeared to be co-operating rather than competing, the example given in the question being local hospitals working together in planning priorities. However, this did not appear to be common to any particular specialties.

The second stage of the study asked trusts about their perceptions regarding the local HA attitude towards competition. The majority of trusts (57.3%) felt that the HA did not encourage competition between trusts while the remainder (42.7%) reported that the local HA was active in supporting competition.

However, when considering the position in relation to local acute and community services, the majority of trusts reported that 'co-ordination' or 'neither co-ordination nor competition' was the approach of the local HA, with only 11% of providers indicating that acute–community competition was supported by the local HA. The latter is an approach which was encouraged by the government in 1994 and 1995.

Explanation

Overall, there has been confusion in national policy. On the one hand, at some points there has been acceptance of co-operative relationships (perhaps, that is, accepting the *consequences* of the market when it produces relative winners and losers who then have to 'co-operate' over local services. Or perhaps it is just accepting that competition does not make much sense, despite the rhetoric, and that providers should be considered as components of a public service rather than as either 'competitors' or 'monopolies'). On the other hand, at other points in time or at other locations, there have been demands from the top for renewed or continual competition.

As a result, local providers and purchasers have not been sure whether to compete or not – and to what extent. The above range of models reflects local adaptation to the game in the light of moving goalposts.

MAJOR RESULTS ON COSTS, QUALITY AND MARKET BEHAVIOUR

The above data and additional conclusions from our case studies suggest that quality is a luxury for most purchasers, despite rhetoric and mission statements, given financial pressures. For hospital providers, worsening quality owing to overwork and underfunding is a real problem, especially in large cities.

As stated at the outset, it is impossible to quote pounds, shillings and pence (or Euros) on the costs of the reforms. A 'ballpark' estimate, however, would be that costs associated with the functions described above have doubled the 'administrative costs' in the NHS – and that these could increase further if fundholding were extended on anything like the current model or arrangements (whether total, standard or limited.)

Costs can of course be justified, even alongside lower quality in major acute hospitals, if improvements elsewhere attributable to the reforms are judged convincingly to outweigh both the management costs and any worsening in services. Such improvements would have to take the form of (for example) new priorities being realised or new services, say in the community, attributable to the reforms and salient in their own right.

Even if the total output of the NHS were less, it could still be argued that some improvements, only realisable through high management costs and pressure on other services, justified this. (This would be the opposite of standard parliamentary defences of the reforms... 'more operations performed' ... etc., etc.)

This would, however, be a strong and controversial claim, especially in an A&E department on a Saturday night. And we do not have evidence that priorities have changed to produce better resource allocation as a result of the reforms. Defenders of the reformers may be on safer ground in stressing higher output of the standard operations. But even here official claims that the reforms have brought these about are suspect. Technological change, including day case work, contributes. Direct political pressure helps. Economy-wide job insecurity may lead to intensified labour in the NHS. But all this is a long way from the market boosting efficiency. The canny old Scots verdict, 'not proven', may be the understated way to conclude.

CONCLUSIONS FROM SURVEYS

It is somewhat surprising to discover such a high mutual dependence between local providers and purchasers when they are trading in such a vast array of services. Arguably this might occur if there are economies of scale and (more importantly) scope to be obtained in health care, since the most efficient provider of one aspect of health care is likely to be the most efficient provider of many aspects of health care. The prediction here, of course, might be that one or two key providers would dominate the entire market and not that a different single provider would dominate with each purchaser.

The other important difference of health care, indicated by our results, as opposed to a traditional market is that of 'location' as part of the product. Otherwise, why is it not the case that particular providers succeed regardless of where they are situated? Thus, while we may find that individuals rely on a restricted range of sources, what dictates these sources is largely the nature and quality of their product, not its location. If we assume that the post-reform NHS market is operating efficiently, how do we account for the geographical element of provision? That is, how do we maintain the concept of a market in health care yet one in which the local provider will always come out on top?

The obvious explanation is that the health-care product contains a number of distinct features, of which location is one. While location does not always dominate over other criteria such as cost and quality, as has already been suggested, it can be a deciding factor in who provides a service to a particular population.

Currently it may be that all providers are broadly similar in terms of the cost and quality of their product, not least due to tightening central control and increased 'squeeze' by a combination of national indicators and tight money. Thus, location becomes an important factor, since it may represent an additional cost to patients and their friends/relatives if travelling is required. Quite simply, local providers dominate HA purchasing, since the combined product that they supply is less costly than their non-local rivals. The reason for this domination is that there is insufficient difference between providers with regard to other aspects of the health-care product to outweigh the travelling costs connected to location. Or rather, travel is determined by clinical criteria and the planning inheritance. This is actually consistent with the concept of competition. If one provider becomes more efficient, there is every incentive for other providers to follow suit. Otherwise, their location would be an insufficient advantage over the greater costs or relatively lower quality of the health-care product they provide with which to gain contracts from their host purchasers.

The conditions for effective competition would break down, however, if 'location' became a dominant cost consideration or was sufficient to alter the definition of the product (i.e. regardless of other features of the product, location will always be the first determinant in the purchasing decision). Thus no matter what the quality of the product and no matter how cheaply you can produce it, the location will always dictate the decision as to whether the purchaser will buy it, i.e. product X at location A is a totally different product from X at location B. In such a situation the market will be restricted within certain geographical boundaries and hence competition will be between a limited number of providers, with the possibility of there being only a single provider and hence no competition.

In contract types, there is a difference between what is used and what is preferred. By and large it is sophisticated block and cost and volume contracts which are preferred but simple and sophisticated block contracts are still used for HAs and cost-per-case (by and large) with GPFHs. The former may be crude ('the old system, with its cash limit, under a new name') and the latter is expensive and unsustainable if generalised.

After the NHS reforms, the provider tends to follow the local HA and aligns what it does to the HA's wants and wishes. This is even more ironic when it is normally the provider which will get the flak if something goes wrong with a patient's care or if waiting times increase or 'rationing' bites. The latter two are (assuming contracts are met) the purchaser's responsibility. But, as the saying goes, the patient can't find the purchaser in the 'phone book'.

Also ironic is the fact that tighter control of local providers by purchasers has followed the institutional separation of purchaser and provider.

A major headache revealed not just by these surveys but the case studies as well is the cost of information. Information systems in most trusts are inadequate for their needs and the cost of staff employed on monitoring has risen considerably over the past few years. This has consequences for other areas. For example, many trusts use inadequate information systems to explain why they have not moved to more activity-based contracts. Yet information to service a functional purchaser/provider split based on sophisticated activity contracts may be a 'bridge too far' for as tightly funded an NHS as we currently have. Even if attainable, greater allocative efficiency plus better alignments of workload and money might leave too little 'real money' for the quantity of care required, due to the costs of information and 'running the system'.

In short, we'd need much more money. But if we had it, we wouldn't need the precision in the first place. The paradox runs as follows. The reformed NHS is costly to run: even where benefits ensue, the costs dig too deep into limited budgets. Yet, if more money were available, it might be better to spend it on patient care, as the benefits of this might be more than the benefits from more complex contracting systems.

CONCLUSIONS FROM CASE STUDIES

It is neither easy nor always sensible to seek exact parallels between national pictures painted by the data analysis (above), on the one hand, and local pictures painted by individual case studies, on the other. The case studies we undertook painted many rich pictures of their own, although confidentiality was required.

It is nevertheless worth pointing out that overall parallels and similar conclusions exist, allowing some aspects of the case studies to be interpreted as putting flesh on the bones of the data survey. Symmetrically, some of the surveys give credibility to local observations made in the case studies. In this regard, some key issues arising from the case studies are summarised below, to compare with results from the national surveys above.

It should be pointed out that the case studies were selected systematically, to reflect national coverage, different types of trust and different types of population covered by health authorities and areas of the country.

The key issues are as follows.

1. There were overwhelming administrative demands as a result of GP fundholding. Most trusts have at least one person dedicated to GP fundholding in the contracts department. The costs of fundholding, and indeed its possibly deleterious effect on services as well, come out of a number of studies. One study (of a combined acute and community trust) led to observations of the advantage of fundholding in being 'close to patients' in the purchase of services, yet also its costs in terms of marketing 'round in circles'.

   Thus, the costs of GP fundholding seem unequivocal while its benefits are equivocal.
2. Consortia of GP fundholders do not necessarily simplify the trust's job. For example, although one might anticipate less complexity if dealing with consortia of GP fundholders rather than individual fundholders as a result of fewer and less diverse contracts, this is not necessarily the case. There are just as many varieties of contract faced by some trusts, in that (although key structures are negotiated *en masse*) each GP prefers to have specific criteria for their practice. Additionally, the GPs' bargaining power is stronger yet the administrative requirements are not necessarily reduced. This can create difficulties for trusts in terms of pressure on management time.

   One study in particular pointed to the fact that consortia may not be internally homogeneous and may have been formed for all sorts of reasons, opportunistic and otherwise. Thus 'economies of scale' in contracting for patients of similar need are not necessarily the result.

   Furthermore, consortia of GP fundholders are often formed to preserve local services rather than to 'make the market work' in a more general sense.
3. Some health authorities are actually returning to block contracts, having moved away from them. Given a shortfall of cash, the health authority believes that extra workload is the problem of the trust. This relates to general observations made in this book about the purchaser/provider split creating a culture of 'buck passing' in many instances. Rather than sharpening up incentives on both sides of the divide, as it were, and ensuring more appropriate and efficient health care, the health authority may have financial power without responsi-

bility for managing the provider. This can have significant perverse effects.

4. The short-term nature of contracting and the annual renegotiation of contracts are frequently seen as ridiculous. It was mentioned on a number of occasions that even rolling contracts effectively involve a new contracting round each year.

   Furthermore, the need for all trusts to 'break even' each year is a major source of inefficiency and rigidity and a boost to short-termism in planning. ('No business would have to operate like that.')

5. Contract negotiations are generally corporate (trust-wide) led, rather than led from individual directorates or specialties (within acute trusts or divisions within community trusts). A typical picture would involve about six or seven meetings each year to agree on contracts, with perhaps another two meetings for conciliation or ironing out of difficulties. Directorates may be consulted but are generally not involved in a formal sense, on grounds of impracticality. A typical picture is that directorates are informed of the result of contractual negotiations and in effect expected to 'come in on line'. Admittedly, intra-trust conflict between directorates and 'the corporate view' could affect future negotiations by board officers of the trust but in many trusts this is a source of frustration for Clinical Directors (doctors) and business managers. They have 'responsibility but not power'; they have to obey contracts in the making of which they have not participated (especially to do with 'waiting list initiatives').
6. GP fundholders' contracts were increasingly precise in some trusts, as health authorities continue to stress (or even return to) broad block contracts. Even this may change, however, and some 'straws in the wind' include the movement to block contracts by certain GP fundholders.
7. The shedding of management posts through central directive means that, although the market still exists, the capacity to make the market sophisticated is diminished. As a result, the administrative costs of the market in general may be retained (although compressed into intensified labour for fewer staff), while the benefits of the market are curtailed or rendered less achievable. One comment from a particular trust: 'Unfortunately a lot of our plans for the future are on hold since we are now at our limit managing where we are ...'.
8. A very typical observation from trusts is that the purchasing function of health authorities is either marginal in its effect or crude and perverse. The net benefit of purchasing must actually be called into question, given the salience and frequency of this observation. Another observation from a number of trusts is that the position is actually getting worse, rather than better. Thus, the problem with 'purchasing' may not be solved by education and changed behaviour,

but rather the difficulty is created by purchasing's structural position in the so-called marketplace. In other words, the purchaser/provider split may have perverse effects and the combination of central directive and limited local flexibility makes purchasing an expensive luxury rather than the linchpin of the system. If health authority purchasing is squeezed between fundholding on the one hand and central directive on the other, then obviously this effect is increased.

9. Trusts may seek special relationships with local GPs as part of their marketing, which may even extend to loans and grants. In other words, loans are made to seek to cement and attract referrals. One trust loaned a local GP group £30 000 to extend their surgery, with the right to call in the loan if referral fell below a certain level. In effect the trust was acting as a bank to the GPs, as allegedly the health authority did not have the money to fund such developments.
10. There will be an increasing need to merge directorates into large divisions given the pressure upon management costs. In the early phase of the reforms, there was often a move to many smaller directorates with high aggregate management costs.
11. It is the dominant perception that most decisions within the NHS are crisis driven rather than increasingly proactive or as part of more innovative policy (or strategy) making.
12. Specialised services are endangered by over-devolved purchasing. One frequent observation is that a national strategy for acute provision is necessary. Different scenarios are possible. It is conceivable that a move to primary care could lead to a concentration of 'standard' secondary provision (through mergers and the like), with a 'knock-on' effect towards concentration of specialist services. In particular specialties, including the treatment of various forms of cancer, concentrated specialised services have been 'audited' as providing the best results. Nevertheless, an alternative scenario is possible, in which specialised services are increasingly provided as part of 'standard' secondary providers.

    In some ways the market is driving the latter, whereas planning is driving the former. This is because secondary providers may seek to market specialised services in order to try to obtain a 'market niche'. Additionally, pricing rules may make purely specialist centres untenable unless specially funded. That is, they require 'bread and butter' work in order to survive financially and do their specialist work.

    All in all, such issues require attention. Rationalisation within, as well as between, sectors may be impossible otherwise. One particular complaint we have found from specialist centres in London is that the 'planning reviews' (following the Tomlinson review and the activities of the London Implementation Group set up to plan specific services and help rationalise provision within London generally) are only one part of a complex politically dominated system. There is also a see-saw between the demands of the market and the interventions of politicians on (arbitrary or opportunistic) 'planning criteria'.

13. The main advantages of the post-reform contracting system are perceived as sharper definition of 'the product' (services) and closer attention to (the purchaser's) demands. If the product is appropriate and if the purchaser represents either legitimate public need or reasonable public expectation, then services may improve.

    Additional advantages are seen as 'an ability to sort out the workforce' (which of course may be seen as a disadvantage by others!) and an ability to devolve responsibility for management to clinicians (which likewise may be a two-edged sword). Quote from one Clinical Director of surgery: 'It would be us that took responsibility for the main purchaser contract ... how else do you explain the total absence of any executive in a major contract [yet presence in all others]?'.
14. Locality purchasing is not the same as protection or nurturing of local services, although often justified as such by elision. The East Cheshire study in particular suggested that, paradoxically, a series of local decisions can render the local service less viable. By implication, larger scale purchasing and commissioning is required to plan the future of specific services. There may be a problem of (lack of) collective action whereby lots of small decisions produce consequences unintended and undesired by all.
15. The planning process is provider driven, with ultimate decisions taken regionally and centrally: this conclusion came from the study of Sheffield and a number of others. Politicians have continually changed their minds about whether the 'quasi-market' means restriction on the market or regulation to increase market forces (the paradox of the 'market as central policy' – the visible fist rather than the invisible hand!). Meanwhile purchasing has been squeezed by relentless intervention by politicians despite their lack of a clear vision.
16. 'Quality' has been about the frills rather than clinical services. A number of chief executives have confidentially commented on declining standards, and indeed crisis, in terms of factors such as 'trolley waits' for emergencies, patients turned away, cancelled elective work, etc.

    Indeed the mushrooming of quality initiatives is arguably in proportion to their need. It is more doubtful whether they can solve the major problems of quality, given existing resources and demands on the system.
17. The purchaser/provider split is used more often as a basis for negotiation between local providers and purchasers rather than as a catalyst for a market. In the case of community services, the health authority

and community trust of necessity have to be close and it varies from place to place as to whether the authority or trust leads in planning and specifying services.

This raises the question as to whether the benefits or costs of the 'split' are greater. Indeed, while management costs are higher than in the days of the integrated health authority in most cases, even the existence of benefits may be in doubt.

Admittedly, most interviewees take the line that 'The purchaser/provider split is here to stay (and good), but the market and the costs associated with the new arrangements are a different story'. This way of interpreting events may itself reflect either pragmatism (the split is now inevitable) or absorption of the new orthodoxy irrespective of the overall balance sheet.

For, especially in an age when rationalisation (i.e. mergers and closures) of hospital services and greater flexibility of services (owing to technological possibilities) are needed, direct control of providers may make more sense, irrespective of ideology or what was instituted through the NHS reforms. That is, negotiating with autonomous trust boards and handling the politics of conflict may make change more difficult. Even the conservatism of local communities when it comes to desirable or inevitable change may be bolstered by the purchaser/provider split. After all, hospitals now have their own boards and 'voice'. That is indeed why the 'decentralisation' of the split is accompanied by the centralisation of regional and national diktat: otherwise, change could not easily be forced.

In framing its health policy in the mid-1990s, the Labour Party was caught on the horns of this dilemma. It seemed too late to reverse the reforms. Secondly, in a mood of caution in the 1997 campaign, it expunged the memory of its rather more radical stance against the reforms in 1992, a stance which was also conservative. Yet it wished to criticise the Conservative government for the 'waste' of the reforms and also the weakening and 'crisis' in the NHS. It was therefore left with the contradiction of claiming, 'Things are terrible; but don't worry, we won't change much'!

The limited institutional changes proposed by Labour included broadening the membership of trust boards (rather than abolishing separate provider boards and reintegrating them). But this ironically makes planning, and managing change, more cumbersome, not less: separate trusts are bedded in to their communities more deeply, as their boards are now 'of the community' rather than business executives.

'Democratisation' makes more sense at the planning tier, if at all. Otherwise, we have the 'problem of the second best': good solutions applied to the wrong institutions. Additionally, reducing management costs may be less likely – as with Labour's agenda for purchasing, which 'democratises' existing arrangements rather than making more thoroughgoing change which is nevertheless administratively manageable. One is reminded of the old adage, 'If you want to get there, I wouldn't start from here'!

18. When things go wrong, it is the providers which get the 'flak' from the public. This was an almost unanimous statement from our interviewees at chief executive and board level. As a result, the purchaser/provider split may diminish rather than increase purchasers' sense of responsibility for services. Problems may therefore become the locus for conflict and buck passing rather than joint working on solutions. The 'new public management' orthodoxy, that policy or planning and implementation or management of provision are best separated, may be shorter lived than its proponents believed.
19. The system of dealing with ECRs may actually have sharpened a problem in the pre-reform NHS. That problem was the perverse incentive that providers might seek patients from outside the locality as the funding formula would reward these more generously. (This occurred when health authority budgets for their own patients were squeezed and the *de facto* costs allowable were less for local patients.) Even then, however, there was no contracting mechanism which made this explicit and often perverse incentives in theory did not become perverse behaviour in practice. Additionally, it was only future targets that were affected, not 'cash up front'. Also, it was not even the provider (let alone the clinical directorate within the provider) but the whole health authority which had its target affected: individual managers (let alone clinicians) did not 'feel' the imperative of the incentive.

    Since the reforms and in particular the purchaser/provider split, ECRs are often funded (at actual cost) more generously than patients under conventional (and especially block) contracts. This process can subvert the health authority's financial control (it has to earmark reserve budgets for ECRs, diminishing money for 'commissioning according to need') and indeed its autonomy as a planner according to need. This state of affairs featured largely in our studies.

    The 'solution', in effect from both main political parties, is to 'abolish' ECRs by deciding in advance what is reimbursed and what is not. But this merely creates a new 'contract' or at least an earmarked (and yet unpredictable) reserve budget. As a result, once again, national regulation squeezes purchasing autonomy. This may be desirable, of course, but if so, why maintain the expensive mechanics of the less and less relevant purchaser/provider split?
20. Finally, there was a split in our interviews between managers who approved of the reforms (overall) and those who saw them as rhetoric

disguising the continuing truth that the NHS is about local services and political domination.

Clinicians are largely (but not exclusively) opposed to the reforms, while resigned to their continuing. They do not see party politics as the source of much change.

Over the three years, scepticism about the reforms grew, maybe in proportion to an increasingly tight central agenda, financial crisis (until just before the 1997 general election) and a growing frustration with year-on-year contracting quarrels and high administrative costs (financial and stress-related, especially as management costs were cut yet their cause retained).

Chapter 5 explores whether or not 'purchasing' (with or without a market) has led to innovative means of making and realising priorities by health authorities and others.

Purchasing: new vintage or just new label?

5

INTRODUCTION

Chapters 1 and 3 have cast doubt on the consistency with which the new institution of purchasing was promoted as the heart of the reforms. Before 1991, the market, the creation of trusts and the operation of the contracting system (as the essence of the purchaser/provider split) took top priority for ministers and therefore managers. Between 1991 and the general election of April 1992, achieving (temporary) stability, to reassure a sceptical public, was the name of the game. After 1992, when the new system was safe as a result of the Conservatives' election victory, it was soon perceived that providers were calling the tune; they had the information and purchasers could at best play around with marginal contracts. So, strong purchasing became the watchword. The same management centres which had spent the Department's millions gearing up trusts (creating their structures and business planning processes; on average, it was estimated that £250 000 per trust were spent on 'communication strategies' alone) were now loosed on purchasers. In the next two years, the then Health Minister Dr Brian Mawhinney's guidance on purchasing would be the hymn-sheet of the faithful (in public). And more was to follow: no sooner had the 'new purchasing' been proselytised as the new rationale for health authorities than it was devolved to GPs. This left health authorities unclear as to their role: was it substantive or regulatory? This uncertainty persists today.

But, before this development, a more fundamental question could be asked. Just what was purchasing? A minimalist definition would be, 'what was left after the providers (trusts) were removed from the health authority'. This would not however go beyond defining the purchaser as one half of the purchaser/provider split – a tautology without function, save to expose circular thinking on the part of policy makers. The old health authority had been responsible for its hospitals and community providers. But it had also planned services within its boundaries and (jointly with the region) sometimes outwith its boundaries, where its residential patients were affected.

How did 'purchasing' differ, other than by translating service plans into market contracts and thereby putting a cap on referrals out of the district, as well as limiting (by implication) care within the district?

The answer was that it did not, with the proviso that the latter tasks are of course big ones. If pre-reform 'underfunding' (i.e. less money than needed to pay for all referred and sought care at existing cost, without long waiting times) was to be 'solved', then it was necessary to ration out the unaffordable and prevent patients getting treatment without a contract. The trouble was, of course, that politicians had instructed the NHS (Management) Executive to deny that that was the intention. This was in truth to deny that there was any point to creating the complex institutions of the reforms! Squaring the circle (of apparent underfunding before the reforms yet no need for rationing after the reforms) was the source of Sir Duncan Nichol's hostage to fortune, when the then chief executive of the NHS told the *Daily Mail* that rationing was not necessary, as the reforms would unleash such productive energy.

On this reading, purchasing was logically about squeezing providers to meet demand at their door, not about priorities, local or national. ('Of course it's not about fancy new priorities, or prevention and promotion, or primary care – it's about hitting providers till they squeal': confidential interview, member of NHS Policy Board, 1994.) Indeed, the subsequent history bears this out: purchasing has been a conduit for central government orders about meeting targets for waiting times, charters without extra cash and the like. Purchasers have, in effect, been mini-ministries and the purchaser/provider split has been co-opted to the task of centralising planning yet decentralising the operational nuts and bolts.

Another reason for purchasing being hailed as a new departure for the NHS is not, this time, another political sleight of hand, but the innocence of many of the new managers who did not know what the old system's planning and resource allocation had done, let alone at its best. Managers who believe the propaganda they are required to read out are the best managers of all, in a system where looking upwards to please the political master had become quickly entrenched as the culture. (This was a nice irony – a very British Stalinism as the result of the Thatcher reforms.)

But this is to jump the gun. To return to the early 1990s, if purchasing were to be the linchpin of the reforms, then the purposes of 'strong purchasing' must be identified. Distinction is often made between the terms 'commissioning' and 'purchasing'. While originally commissioning (deriving from the naval term) referred to the bringing on stream of a new hospital, it is now (to the extent it is distinguished from purchasing) a kind of hybrid between identifying priorities and planning to meet them, on the one hand, and working with providers to ensure that the identified objectives are met, on the other. Purchasing, as one might expect, is more to do with buying services identified in the commissioning process. Thus there is a continuum from large-scale planning, through commissioning, through purchasing, to contracting, and then to monitoring of the contract and repeating those elements of the process as necessary.

THE OLD NHS

In the pre-reform NHS, from 1976 onwards resources were allocated to districts (via regions, from the Department of Health) and they were intended to allocate these resources to meet health needs within their district. Alongside this, however, lay a planning process which did not just involve districts but also regions. As a result, the planning process might assume that patients would move from district to district in pursuit of the most relevant location for their services.

In other words there was a resource allocation methodology on the one hand and a separate planning methodology on the other.

As a result, some technical problems arose in reconciling the implications of the two different methodologies and strategies which flowed from them. When patients flowed from one district to another, the way the money reimbursed the recipient district meant that, for similar cases, the formula attributed a different sum of money for inflowing patients from that which was allocated by the recipient district for its local patients. This maybe did not matter too much. After all, what the formula implied and what the district actually got from its region might not be the same thing. Also, in those days, the commercialism of the market was not dominant in the NHS (indeed did not exist at all) and therefore those who made the financial decisions as to whether to treat patients or not, and how to treat them, were not really swayed by where the patient came from.

Nevertheless, the system had its disadvantages. Firstly, the region adjusted district's allocations to cope with such flows, such that what the district was left with for those patients treated locally might not be adequate to meet the potential caseload. This of course was a problem of the total finance, rather than of the system of planning or resource allocation used. Next, there was no guarantee that, when the formula moved money from one district to another, that district would use the money in the wisest way possible. In other words, hospitals responsible for 'generating the extra work' could not be guaranteed to receive the money, unless the good management of the district ensured that this was so. Finally, given that the formula was used to create targets yet those targets were not necessarily implemented quickly, 'earning extra money' on the part of districts or hospitals did not necessarily translate into extra money in practice quickly enough.

THE REFORMS

This was the situation which led to the diagnosis of the NHS's problem by Alain Enthoven (1985) and his advocacy of an internal market. It is now history as to how, why and after what period of time and consideration of alternative options the internal market was eventually adopted through the NHS reforms. Nevertheless, the internal market created problems which are arguably sharper and worse than those originally diagnosed in the old NHS. In line with our attempt to look at who takes decisions and who has the power, let us review the reformed NHS.

Firstly, money now flowed to health authorities (and GP fundholders) who would purchase directly on behalf of their patients. As well as perverse incentives which develop in practice as a result of this situation (many of which are due to the purchaser/provider split), one major issue arises. This is the fact that there is no longer free referral (without consideration of finance) around the system. In the old NHS, after the system had been planned, GPs were free to refer around the system. Now, 'purchasing' has been developed. Even before one considers the purchaser/provider split and interactions between purchasers and providers, it is important to note that in the old NHS overt purchasing did not exist, whereas in the reformed NHS it does.

Purchasing means fundamentally that contracts are placed with providers and that somehow referrals and caseload/workload in the system must be rendered compatible with these contracts. Where this does not occur, 'extracontractual referrals' have to be paid for, either absorbed by the purchaser or the provider. The major implication of having such 'purchasing' is that incentives are set up whereby cases reimbursed, or reimbursed generously, through such purchasing are welcome whereas other cases are not.

Another argument for purchasing was that, in the context of limited budgets, it could allow communities and GPs (not the same!) to have more power *vis-à-vis* hospital clinicians and 'specialists' generally. It was also argued that the GP is nearer to the patient than the hospital doctor. As a result, giving power to GPs will increase consumer power (if it is acceptable to call a patient a consumer in the first place!).

There is a large paradox here, however. In the old system, when planning worked as it was intended to, hospitals were designed to cope with predicted need on the basis of relevant information for their relevant areas, with assumptions taken into account (for example) as to how far it was reasonable to expect patients to travel. Once such hospitals and community facilities were created, GPs could refer to them as they wished and money flowed around the system with adjustments being made to districts' (health authorities') allocations as described above. In other words, there was not purchasing, in the sense of restrictions on flows as a result of financial allocations made by purchasers. There was reimbursement within available resources, i.e. within the system which had been created.

This right has been removed. Except in the case of fundholding general practitioners (who in any case have to work within cash limits and, to the extent that they become the dominant force in the system, will have to do the 'dirty work' of health authorities), referrals have to be in line with contracts.

As a result, to prevent GPs (of the non-fundholding variety) rebelling openly or finding their rights wholly undermined, the rhetoric is all about 'involving GPs in purchasing decisions.' This is presented as involving new rights for GPs. It is in fact developing minor rights to replace the major right which has been removed, albeit a major right which was often exercised conservatively and/or without input into the broader planning of services.

To put it in a nutshell: in the old system, planning was done and GPs were then free to refer. Whether or not GPs fed into such planning in the first place was an open question. (The cultural change to involve GPs and patients more generally is less to do with the market or the NHS reforms than with changing power relationships and ideologies within society as a whole.) A further paradox to keep in mind was that no sooner had health authorities been given the responsibility for 'strong purchasing' than it was taken away from them, by 'empowering' GPs for the above reasons. Again, policy was too transitory to allow either certainty or capacity building by health authorities.

In the post-reform NHS, planning in the broadest sense is nevertheless still undertaken centrally, with regional offices and indeed the Department of Health – often acting through political instructions (for example, to save sensitive hospitals) – taking the key decisions as to which hospitals expand, which contract, which close and which merge. Then, and only then, can GPs be involved in the contracting process, to which they are then bound. In other words, GPs probably do not plan; they may or may not be involved in purchasing; and their rights of free referral are removed.

To summarise:

- Old NHS:
  1. planning (whether or not 'participatory');

2. free referral by GPs but some financial disincentives to effective allocations at the micro level.

- Post-reform NHS:
  1. planning, but now covert, undertaken centrally by region(al offices) and the Department of Health;
  2. purchasing decisions taken by health authorities and fundholders (maybe involvement in health authority decision making by non-fundholding GPs and indeed fundholders also; maybe not). Such purchasing is dependent on the facilities created in planning although of course it may provide guidance for future planning, by expressing preferences. In this aspect, 'purchasing' is just a technical component of planning;
  3. *not* free referral, except within cash-limited budgets by GP fundholders.

DECENTRALISING PURCHASING: GPS AND LOCALITIES

An evolving policy concerning commissioning and purchasing has thus been to decentralise it by involving GPs and so-called localities. For the Conservatives, before they lost the election in 1997, fundholding was the preferred option and, while not obligatory, regional offices had performance targets and reviews based on percentages of GPs who had become fundholders. It appeared to be voluntary at practice level and mandatory at authority level and above! Paradoxically, it was the rapid 'widening and deepening' of fundholding (more fundholders, holding budgets for more services) which made it necessary to co-ordinate fundholders' choices with health authority and provider choices. Extension of fundholding was to a large part a political choice: if fundholding was bedded in, Labour could not easily abolish it. Co-ordinating fundholders with health authorities in the planning process was necessary if planning were not to be anarchic (see Chapters 6 and 7).

The sting in the tail for fundholders is, of course, that the attraction in the first place may be the promise of freedom. If that is bureaucratised, the attraction may soon fade. One survey as early as 1994 suggested that 40% of first-wave fundholders opposed fundholding and had 'gone for it' because there might be advantages in getting in quickly. This makes some sense: if nearly all GPs are fundholders, then financial carrots soon disappear, unless cash limiting is abolished. The then chairman of the BMA's HSMC Committee, John Chawner, described incentives to fundholders as a 'bung' in 1994.

One means of involving fundholders in authority planning is to generalise the opportunity to all GPs. Then they do not seem to be 'singled out' for 'reining in'. There are various means of doing this: involving GPs in health authority decisions; consulting various GP practices when taking such decisions; devolving authority decision making, in part or in whole, to localities, in which GPs participate; or devolving decisions to GP practice-based units of the authority's territory.

Labour, for its part, came close to government policy, although 'harder' on fundholding. In December 1996, Chris Smith, the latest in a long line of Shadow Health Spokesmen, stated that fundholders could continue if they had the consent of their non-fundholding colleagues in the locality and were involved in commissioning by locality, feeding in (one assumes) to the health authority plan. This was a softening of the previous abolitionist line. After their election victory, however, Labour halted extensions of fundholding, while setting out regulations which sought to prevent fundholders' patients having advantages in terms of waiting time.

In practice, there was less difference between the parties on this issue than met the eye. The new orthodoxy, of GP as hero, now ran deep. For Labour, of course, sounding GP friendly in general was a means of diffusing fundholder hostility in the run-up to 1997 and after.

But a lot of questions remain unanswered. Why GPs and not nurses as community representatives? Is the policy about empowering communities, or (more likely) giving GPs budgets and therefore reining in their expectations as to what the NHS can provide (as well as hoping GPs can 'do it more cheaply')?

Participation by all GPs on behalf of the community may not produce the best results in terms of greater equalisation of health status (defined as equality of result, rather than simply equality of opportunity to participate in planning). That is, devolution of budgets or indicative budgets to GPs may produce less equity, when a very good formula is used, than 'equal resources to all'. But even such a formula will be allocated to over-small populations, producing over time variations in need with which rigid, overdevolved allocations cannot cope.

There is a trade-off between allocating resources to small areas on the basis of need (adjusting for greater medical need through resource allocation formula) and ensuring that resources are centralised enough to allow effective planning. Locally held resources may mean local accountability but also inability of providers to predict on a stable enough basis where the money is coming from and planning budgets which are too small to allow spread of risk over time.

As a result, it makes sense to allocate resources to health authorities on the basis of need; to involve GPs and representatives of localities in using resources, certainly, but in a lean and efficient manner; and to ensure that regions (above the district level) have a role in adjusting resource allocations in line with desired flows.

Arguably, GPs and localities ought *not* to have decision-making powers so much as a say in, or contribution towards, such a decision-making power. To put it simply: a GP practice in an affluent area within a district should not have the same rights to spend the same amount of money as a GP practice in a less affluent area if the health need is greater in the latter area. A simple 'head count' of GPs on the question of priorities can be misleading if the aim is to address health needs in an equitable and progressive manner. There would be a danger of 'undoing' past resource reallocation in search of equity.

It can of course be argued that holding resources at a higher level (such as the regional level) may allow them to be allocated equitably and with stability, but this will fail to ensure that the areas, localities or indeed patients on whose behalf they are allocated will use them. It could be argued that devolution of actual purchasing power (to, for example, GP fundholders) could ensure that they can actually buy the services on behalf of the relevant patients and ensure that it is the relevant patients who get them. There is some truth in this, in theory. In practice, however, ensuring that the needy use services is often something that can only be achieved through wider social activity, sponsored from a higher tier rather than through precise allocations to local budget holders.

COMMISSIONING FOR EQUITABLE HEALTH GAIN

The reality is that policy on commissioning for health gain was national. Devolution of choice to local purchasers was marginal. This is not an implied criticism of government policy. It is inevitable that, if the concept of the National Health Service is to retain legitimacy, there will be national decisions as to priorities and national applications of methodologies for prioritisation and even 'rationing'. What was confusing was the distance between reality and rhetoric. The rhetoric implied local choice by purchasers. While the National Health Service has always varied across the country (and not just due to historical imbalances of resources), local choice will be limited if the NHS uses robust methodologies for making priorities; allocates resources according to a formula which measures need (admittedly a contested concept); and holds purchasers accountable for outcomes. Genuine devolution (if, for example, Sheffield Health Authority makes decisions entirely different to neighbouring districts) will always cause problems. Firstly, supra-health authority planning at regional and national levels is required to ensure appropriate rationalisation and provision of services. Secondly, accountability to Parliament, and more particularly to the NHS executive and to auditing agencies, will in practice ensure greater uniformity than this. Thirdly, the long-term consequence of genuinely local choice could be the demise of central funding and central resource allocation, as such resource allocation gauges need according to universal or national criteria. Local choice implies local revenue generation. This could still leave scope for some form of equalisation between poor and rich areas, but such is a minefield (Paton, 1995).

Currently, there is much public disquiet about locally based 'rationing', such as exists. It is therefore important to find the appropriate balance between national and local priority setting when it comes to commissioning and purchasing. Under the Conservatives national policy focused broadly upon individual causes of ill health and therefore targeted individual behaviour. This was the broad thrust of the *Health of the Nation* strategy from 1992 onwards. Although research was later commissioned to consider 'health variations' (the then Conservative government could not bring itself to use the term 'inequalities'), this was a research agenda rather than a policy agenda and it targeted 'micro' variations within districts rather than the 'macro' causes of ill health and health inequalities.

A criticism of policy therefore is not that it was national but that it was inadequately comprehensive. The Black Report of 1980 was rejected by the then incoming Conservative government, having been commissioned by the previous Secretary of State. The so called 'blacker report' (Whitehead, 1987) pointed to the worsening of trends and literature reviewed below suggests that things were getting worse in terms of health inequalities by the 1990s. The Labour government of 1997 returned to the issue of inequalities with a new Minister for Public Health, Tessa Jowell.

Whether one is concerned with the maximisation of health gain or the greater equalisation of health status or indeed a policy which tackles objectives within both aspirations, it is now a commonplace in research that a whole range of social factors determine mortality rates, morbidity rates and health generally. Indeed, one of the reasons why the national regulation and control of 'local purchasing' is so tight is that, currently, the NHS is expected to provide a disproportionately high share of the general attack upon ill health. It is expected to provide the hospitals for cure (albeit decreasingly for care); various non-hospital means of care; and the whole gamut of aspirant policy for prevention and promotion. Multi-agency activity is paid lip service and little more (through 'Healthy Alliances', in terms of working with local authorities and voluntary organisations).

We are expecting the NHS to 'carry the can' for deficiencies in other social (and indeed economic) policy, and this means that local leeway is limited. When one also accepts the fact that a whole range of targets were also set for secondary care in the sense of 'waiting list' initiatives, charters and various targets based on national indicators, it is not surprising that there was strong central pressure directing the use of remaining budgets. This is also a trend detected in our analysis and commented upon in a number of our case studies.

Broadly speaking, policy within the National Health Service for prevention and promotion between 1992 and 1997 sought to attack various individual causes of ill health, but otherwise was limited. Politically speaking, there has long been a section of the Left which is 'anti-doctor and anti-hospital'. To this lobby, diverting resources away from hospital care is appealing, as well as to the cost cutting Right in politics, which wishes both to limit the total NHS budget and yet to make the NHS carry the can more and more, while other social budgets are cut. Thus there is pressure on budgets for both primary and secondary care.

Unless on utopian assumptions, investing more in genuine primary care (prevention and promotion, not just secondary care in the community) is not likely to diminish the demand or need for acute care. Even a utopian assumption of the effectiveness of widespread health promotion (targeting social as well as individual causes) might well lead to a longer term scenario where death and disease are postponed in the lifecycle, but where the need for subsequent complex care is increased, not decreased. A concept of 'substitute morbidity and mortality' has some relevance here (Netherlands Ministry of Health, Welfare and Sports, 1995).

Attacking inequalities in health – which is also likely to increase health gain, as we are far from the point at which the trade-off between the two becomes salient – thus requires a wide range of social and economic policy. In the meanwhile, we must accept that the National Health Service needs to focus upon secondary care to a greater degree than many advocates of our 'primary care-led NHS' admit. Other agencies must take their share of a genuine 'primary' strategy for health care and, additionally, social care cannot reasonably be defined out of the NHS unless it is accounted for through other agencies or through new financing mechanisms.

The next sections review the potential contribution of purchasing in two realms – addressing health inequalities and involving localities. These may be considered as 'tracer' policies addressing outcomes and processes, respectively. That is, if purchasing is to tackle significant outcomes, equity (and particularly meeting health needs to reduce inequality) is a good area to investigate: if it can't make an impact here, its pretensions as regards outcomes must be lowered. Similarly, involving local communities is a good 'tracer' for purchasing's ability to achieve improved process, i.e. procedural quasi-rights for localities. Again, if it cannot deliver here, its pretensions may be seen as just that – pretensions.

A CHALLENGE FOR THE NEW 'PURCHASING AS MEETING NEED': ADDRESSING INEQUALITY

Considering inequalities in health is instructive for the purpose of considering whether 'the new purchasing' is up to the job of tackling them. That is, tackling inequality is a 'tracer condition' for the effectiveness of purchasing in achieving desired outcomes.

The persistence of inequalities in health is of particular significance when set against the provision of health care services since the inception of the NHS. As Townsend *et al.* highlight:

> Inequalities in health are of concern to the whole nation and represent one of the biggest possible challenges to the conduct of government policy ... Britain [has] failed to match the improvement in health observed in some other countries and has acknowledged the relationship of this to persistent internal inequalities of health. (Townsend *et al.*, 1988, p1)

One of the principles on which the NHS was founded was that of equity, particularly in relation to the financial status of the individual (i.e. 'to divorce the care of health from questions of personal means or other factors irrelevant to it': Cartwright and O'Brien, 1976). Associations between people's social position and their health status had long been recognised (in the 19th century, for example, reports on the 'labouring classes' highlighted that those who were poor experienced a higher incidence of illness and disease than those who were rich (Poor Law Commissioners Report, 1842)), and it was envisaged that with equitable health care available to all, free at the point of delivery, the health of the nation would improve and inequalities in health gradually diminish.

Whilst it may be argued that the overall absolute health of the British population has significantly improved during this century (since the average life expectancy is now 74 for men and 79 for women compared to 45.5 and 49 at the turn of the century), this general increase masks relative inequalities in health that remain within the population as a whole (Wilkinson, 1989). There is now considerable evidence to suggest that in many countries (including the UK) there are differences in health between both different social groups and different geographical regions. Such inequalities in health are particularly apparent in relation to occupational class, ethnicity and gender (DHSS, 1980; Haynes, 1991; MacIntyre, 1986; Townsend *et al.*, 1988; Whitehead, 1987). In the 1990s, for example:

> Poor people [still] die younger than people who are rich; they are more likely to suffer from most of the major 'killer' diseases; and they are more likely to suffer from chronic long standing illnesses ... [and] middle aged men commonly show rates of chronic disease 40 to

50 per cent higher in the lowest compared with the highest social groups. (Nettleton, 1995, p160; Whitehead, 1992, p291).

Much attention has been given to the social pattern of inequalities in health within the past decade in particular (DHSS, 1980; Townsend *et al.*, 1988; Whitehead, 1987). The focus of this debate has centred predominantly on differences in mortality, morbidity and service use between certain groups within the population, the extent of these differences, their variation and causation. Inequalities in health are, according to Whitehead (1992), significant in that they highlight the unfavourable health status of certain sections of the population and are important because they may be unnecessary and avoidable, and highlight a potential decline in human economic potential (Moon and Gillespie, 1995). Furthermore, given that both the health needs and health status of subgroups within a population are potentially diverse, the presence of such inequalities has possible ramifications for both health services provision and strategy. This section briefly outlines the main associations between social position and health and illness and discusses some of the implications of this for service policy.

Evidence of health inequalities in relation to occupational class is probably the most widely documented feature of social differences in the health of populations. Official statistics for England and Wales clearly highlight that disparities exist in mortality and morbidity rates between people of differing social and economic backgrounds throughout the duration of their life. For example, in 1987, children who were born to parents in the Registrar General's social classes IV and V (semiskilled manual and unskilled manual) had a 148% greater chance of dying during their first week of life than children born to parents in social classes I and II (professional and intermediate). Whilst such inequalities are apparent within many European countries, Whitehead points to the reduction in infant mortality between socioeconomic groups in Denmark and Sweden as evidence that the differing mortality rates are not necessarily the result of a 'natural law'. Since the 1930s, for example, Sweden has reduced what was a threefold difference between the infant mortality rates of different occupational groups to approximately 10% (Whitehead, 1992, p306). Furthermore, within the UK during the late 1980s, the mortality rates for adults in social class V were approximately twice as high as those in social class I (OPCS, 1986) and during the period 1989–90 the prevalence rates for long-standing illness within the population were 291 per 1000 for those in the professional classes and 478 per 1000 for those in unskilled occupations (CSO, 1992).

The most comprehensive studies of health inequalities within England and Wales (DHSS, 1980; Whiteheasd, 1987) both suggest that a clear class gradient exists in relation to mortality and morbidity within the population. That is to say, the lower the occupational class, the higher the incidence of mortality (and this is especially true in relation to infant mortality rates). Furthermore, given that lifestyle factors such as income and housing are largely related to occupation (and therefore class position), patterns of mortality are also linked to such variables. As Wilkinson (1986) highlights, if income alone is considered, the correlation with mortality may be even stronger and as Townsend *et al.*'s (1988) study of health and deprivation illustrated, of the four elements of deprivation considered (housing tenure, unemployment, car ownership and overcrowding), car ownership was found to be a particularly salient indicator of health differences. These reviews of mortality and morbidity within the population also illustrated that class gradients in mortality vary when considering the cause of death, and similar trends are apparent when considering patterns of morbidity.

Whilst there is some debate as to whether the classification of the population according to the Registrar General's social class categories is an accurate and appropriate measure by which to analyse the health status of the population (Carr-Hill, 1987; Illsley and Le Grand, 1987; Saunders, 1993), the classification does correlate fairly well with such factors as education and income and remains one of the principal standards by which health status is assessed.

Given that social classes are not evenly distributed throughout the UK, it is not surprising to find differences in the health status of local populations. Much of the literature of the 1980s, however, identified the differences between north and south in the UK. From 1979–83 data, death rates were highest in Scotland, followed by the north and north west regions of England, and were lowest in the south east of England and East Anglia, confirming the long established north–south gradient.

In 1980 the Black Report (DHSS, 1980) concluded, after a careful review of many studies, that while genetic and cultural or behavioural explanations played their part in affecting inequalities in health, the predominant explanation lay in the material circumstances and conditions of people's lives, summarised by the concept of material deprivation.

Some types of disease/illness are, of course, genetically transmitted and it has been argued that natural selection acts as a predisposition to health status and therefore impacts on an individual's life chances (and social class position). However, the natural/biological explanation for inequalities in health, whilst having some impact on the patterning of health, has generally been discounted as a major cause of differential health status between subgroups within the population. Although, as Wadsworth (1986) found in his study of ill health amongst young men, those who experienced serious illness tended to fall down the social scale by the age of 26 (see also Illsley, 1955; Meadows, 1961; Stern,

1983), it has also been highlighted that such movement between the classes is, by and large, too small to have a significant effect on the total figures (Wilkinson, 1986). Furthermore, it is argued that this effect is typically confined to younger men as opposed to older adults (Fox and Shewry, 1988). The selection argument (that healthier people move up the social hierarchy and those who are unhealthy move down), promoted by Stern (1983), primarily views health as a fixed or genetic entity, largely independent of an individual's social and economic circumstances. However, the plausibility of such an approach relies on the extent to which people can insulate their health status from their material conditions during the course of their lifetimes and hence such an argument is difficult to prove both practically and methodologically. As Blane (1985) comments, the methodological problems which surround such studies highlight that 'at best, [health plays] a minor role in mobility' and therefore the marked inequalities in health which are evident within the UK population cannot be explained by natural/biological selection alone.

Health is known to be affected by material circumstances and by patterns of behaviour. Diet, smoking, exercise, etc. may all be relevant to the health status of particular groups (Blaxter, 1990). Accordingly, therefore, might health differences that are apparent between the classes simply be a result of differences in the culture and behaviour of various groups? This could lead to a situation whereby the 'blame' for ill health is placed on individuals (as a result of smoking or poor diet, for example), although such an approach ignores the many and varied reasons as to why individuals choose to adopt particular health behaviours. A healthy diet may, for example, be more expensive than what is regarded as an unhealthy diet. Smoking and drinking may be perceived by those who adopt such behaviour as strategies for coping with particularly difficult circumstances. The perceived costs of such behaviour may be lower, due to different values and more fatalism about life, and the (short-term) benefits may be relatively higher. Furthermore, if such behaviours are responsible for the differential mortality rates between the classes, one would expect to find the differences in mortality wholly due to illnesses and disease associated with these health behaviours. However, for all the major causes of death there are social class differences in mortality rates (Kaplan, 1985). Differences in health behaviour and inequalities in health may therefore be closely related to an individual's material circumstances.

Material deprivation, whilst relative to the social and economic norms of any society, has come to be regarded as a particularly significant factor in explaining inequalities in health. Those subgroups within the population who live in poor housing or in conditions detrimental to their health (such as damp conditions, poor diet, overcrowding) experience higher mortality and morbidity rates than those with more advantaged material circumstances.

Additionally, working conditions may also impact on inequalities in health. Lung cancer and emphysema are, for example, related to working conditions even when smoking is controlled for (RUHBC, 1989, p105). Whilst the total impact (either direct or indirect) of income on health status requires further study, the principal conclusion which may be drawn from recent research in this area suggests that material circumstances have a particularly dominant impact on inequalities in health.

The evidence for inequalities in health and the explanation by reference to material deprivation advocated by the Black Report (DHSS, 1980) and The Growing Health Divide (Whitehead, 1987) was not, however, supported by Conservative government policy. Rather, as Moon and Gillespie (1995) note, 'Successive governments throughout the 1980s and 1990s have particularly targeted the importance of individual responsibility for health behaviour'. Whitehead comments that 'There just has not been a recognisable national effort to tackle inequalities in health' (Whitehead, 1987, p350). The general ethos of recent government policy has not been responsive to this problem. In particular, little has been done to address the extensive inequalities in income, opportunity and resource distribution that underpin the distribution of health and ill health.

Following the NHS reforms, attention focused predominantly on policies that promoted the discipline of the market in health provision in an effort to increase the efficiency and effectiveness of the service rather than equity. Critics such as the BMA and members of the RCS have expressed concern that this may, in turn, lead to greater inequalities (Whitehead, 1994). Indeed, as Whitehead's recent study highlights, the inequalities between the health of adults in differing socioeconomic groups are increasing.

Major social and economic changes have also, over the last decade, placed ever-increasing demands on health service resources as a result of continued high levels of unemployment, a growing proportion of families experiencing poverty (Goodman and Webb 1994), more single parent families and the continuing growth in the proportion of elderly people in the population. These groups have higher than average health risks and represent an unequal burden on health services.

Accordingly, within the confines of a limited budget for health-care purchasing, such factors should by implication play a major part in determining the purchasing plans of health authorities. But if they do, other needs and demands may go by default. In practice, (central) advice and instructions to purchasers have taken the form of advocacy of 'inter-agency' action, such as 'Healthy Alliances' with local government, other central and local agencies and community and voluntary groups. These may produce worthwhile initiatives in themselves, as may 'joint planning' generally between the NHS and local government, the latter incidentally going back to the 1970s even as official policy (and before then unofficially).

The problem is that the NHS budget is then used as a surrogate for the whole social policy budget, in seeking to tackle inequality. Alongside this, the new purchasing is intended as a conduit for governmental priorities and strategies, such as *The Health of the Nation* (which overtly avoided inequalities). In 1994, inequality made a disguised comeback as a concern, via the Chief Medical Officer's Working Group on Health Variations (sic). Such variations were to be tackled as local variations, however: seeking to tackle them thus might be difficult in the absence of national policy and, more conceptually, might not diminish national variations even if successful.

If the new purchasing is (against the rhetoric) really about furnishing agencies to do the centre's bidding, then it could be used strategically if central policy was concerned with inequality. Then, of course, it is planning renamed. If, however, it is about local choice and local decisions as to priorities, then by definition it cannot be about addressing national, regional or class-based inequalities; nor can it be about addressing local inequalities systematically if it is up to local purchasers whether or not these are a priority! And incidentally, if local choices are to have local legitimacy, they cannot be simply the choices of quangocrats.

PURCHASING: NEEDS ASSESSMENT OR LOCAL CONSULTATION?

So, if purchasing is to be about local choices, what in turn does that mean? And how can it also be about needs assessment? Can the circle be squared? Let us now explore in more detail the issues about local communities and GPs, raised earlier. As stated above, this is a useful 'tracer' for purchasing's ability more generally to promulgate improved processes in procuring services. It would be nice to know which issues 'localities' highlight as priorities. Do they include inequality? Are they consistent? Is there a common pattern across the country? Who dominates local policy? As yet, however, local consultation (in any meaningful sense) is in its infancy, despite ideas as to how to proceed (Coote and Hunter, 1996). Tracing *how* authorities are beginning to consult the public is more feasible.

The term 'needs assessment' has taken on a technical air, as if it provides a value-neutral means of assessing needs within limited budgets.

Needs assessment is what it says it is – the assessment of needs! There are rival means of so doing and different methodologies for assessing need within the NHS budget. Given current levels of expenditure on the welfare state (and other expenditure), choices within health programmes may involve major choices between broad priorities. Our own evidence and other recent evidence on purchasing suggests that, for understandable reasons, purchasers are unable to provide magical local solutions to such problems – and therefore they seek national guidance.

Furthermore, 'needs assessment' by experts may produce different priorities from those established by consulting people generally. One particular means of 'assessing need', of course, is to involve local publics. To some extent this is buck passing. If there are hard choices to be made, they can be legitimised by persuading the people that they have made them themselves. A less cynical interpretation of the policy is that it is a necessity and that therefore it is worthwhile to allow local choice where possible. There are different means of conceptualising as well as implementing local choice. Another component of our research sought to consult purchasing organisations as to how they engage with the issue of 'listening to local voices'. (Only later will research be possible on what priorities were gradually established, if any, across the nation.)

The NHS Executive document *Guidance in Priorities and Planning for the NHS 1995/96* (EL (95)68) gave as one of its six medium-term priorities, 'Give greater voice and influence to users of NHS services and their carers in their own care, the development and definition of standards set for NHS services locally and the development of NHS policy both locally and nationally'.

The criteria of success to be used for evaluating progress included:

> [Health authorities should have] a strategic plan for, and should be engaged in, systematic and continuing communication and consultation with local people ... in respect of the development of local services, purchasing plans, specific health issues and health promotion as appropriate ... should be able to demonstrate how consultation and dialogue has influenced the development, planning and purchasing of services: and feedback to local people and groups on the outcome of consultation.

Such sentiments are not new in the provision of health services. Almost 20 years ago the Alma Ata Declaration (1978) issued by the WHO and UNICEF in Geneva stated, 'The people have the right and duty to participate individually and collectively in the planning and implementation of their healthcare'. The latest framework within which participation is described stems from EL (92)1 *Local Voices*.

THE SURVEY

The percentage of responding purchasers who had a defined individual responsible for developing work connected to local voices was 69%. The identified individuals came from a range of professional backgrounds and ranged from director level through to more junior posts.

A core area of the questionnaire was based on a taxonomy of the possible topics within a Local Voices strategy. The classification was taken from a speech by the then Minister for Health, Dr Brian Mawhinney, given at a national purchasing conference in Birmingham on April 13th 1994: 'I want to concentrate on an issue which is central to the success, credibility and legitimacy of purchasers – that is, the involvement of local people in purchasing'.

He went on to describe a review undertaken in January 1994 of actions to involve local people and broke down the concept of involvement into a number of different processes:

1. knowing local people's perceptions, preferences and experiences of health services;
2. establishing local legitimacy for priorities and purchasing intentions, making every effort to consult and take account of people's views;
3. consulting before decisions are made with a clear picture of what can and can't be negotiated and why;
4. modifying plans 'perhaps in the short term' to gain public support;
5. ensuring a preliminary and then formal process which demonstrates changes as a result of consultation;
6. forming a clear communication strategy which informs and improves public knowledge.

Based on a modification of this listing, purchasers were asked to rate the level of importance given to each aspect. The levels ranged from 4 as most important, to 1 as least important. The results are as described in Table 5.1.

The consideration of other data from the questionnaire enables a clearer picture of the progress in public involvement and puts the commitment to action into a more practical frame.

Respondents were asked to sort the various techniques used to gain public involvement under four distinct purposes, giving each a rating which referred to the level of response from 1 (no response) to 4 (substantial response). The four purposes were:

1. gathering public opinion on current services
2. consultation on purchasing plans
3. informing and educating
4. feeding back the results of consultation.

Table 5.1. Types of involvement.

Topic area	Usage (% of purchasers)	Importance (Scale of 1–4)
Knowing local preferences	69	4
Prior consultation	69	4
Communication strategy	72	4
Gaining agreement	66	3
Explaining what can and cannot be done	38	1
Process for change	55	2
Feedback	72	3

Further classification showed which techniques were considered to be most successful in fulfilling their purpose – again on a scale from 1 to 4 (most successful). Very few techniques were scored at level 4. Of these, few were in common use, as shown in Table 5.2.

From this small sample of purchasing organisations, there are some key questions which need to be answered.

- Are techniques being used which are relatively simple to organise, but not necessarily believed to be successful in their outcomes?
- How much energy is being put into processes which are not considered to be successful – or should this read 'How much lip service are we paying to this process?'.
- Is enough thought being given to evaluating current activity and learning from best practice?

It is a fair conclusion that, at present, consultation with the health authority's public and local publics within the boundaries of the Health Authority is just that – consultative. The more innovative health authorities seek to ask more salient questions about overall priorities, but again

Table 5.2. Use of 'successful' means.

Technique	*Use*	*Rating (%)*
Questionnaire	Gathering opinions	11.4
Focus groups	Gathering opinions	7.1
User groups/patients	Gathering opinions	7.1
Local existing groups	Even spread of uses	5.7

the national policy imperatives prevent these from being a strategic input into health authority planning.

Communication of the inevitable is a major form of public communication! 'Educating' the public on both resource constraints and possible hard choices within these resources would perhaps make a suitable characterisation of the policy 'local ears' rather than Local Voices.

INVOLVING COMMUNITIES OR INVOLVING GPS?

It was pointed out, in comparing the old NHS with the post-reform NHS, that a central element of the change consists in the move from free referral by GPs to services they had probably not had much of a say in planning, to a system where GPs (non-fundholders) are generally mandated by contracts but therefore expect a say in commissioning the services. Fundholders may also expect a say in health authority policy, as was obvious in a survey carried out in Anglia and Oxford Region (Harrison, 1996).

As with consultation with patients (consumers) or citizens, the danger is that mechanisms for involvement are both bureaucratic and costly. Direct consumer sovereignty would have transactions costs; 'participative purchasing' of the sort described above has high management costs. It is therefore important to ensure that input by GPs into the process of commissioning services is conducted at an appropriate level.

Traditionally, prior to the reforms, health authorities would have limited input from a GP representative. This was, of course, a far cry from GP-dominated purchasing. Returning to the continuum which runs from planning through commissioning/purchasing through contracting to monitoring and feedback, our research suggests that there is a failure to determine even at a basic conceptual level what 'input by GPs' means. This applies both to the GPs and to the health authority boards responsible for involving them.

Perhaps inevitably, the focus was upon emerging processes and structures rather than research-based policy. It is simply not known yet which methods work or which are associated with improved outcomes. Again, the infusion of political control into local strategy (and reaction by local management to political control) suggests that initiatives may be either politically reactive or reflecting local 'political' circumstances (such as the balance between fundholders and non-fundholders) rather than in accordance with some would-be gold standard or ideal model.

With the development up to 1997 of GP fundholding and the extension to 'total fundholding' whereby nearly all services are purchased by GP fundholders, there is a range of options for GP involvement in purchasing. This extends from total purchasing by GP fundholders, with real budgets, organised into large consortia of fundholders; individual or smaller groups of GP fundholding; what is called locality purchasing with devolved budgets; locality purchasing with nominal budgets; input by GPs (by various mechanisms) into health authority commissioning; through to 'centralised' health authority commissioning. It is important to stress that these models are neither all-inclusive nor mutually exclusive.

Locality purchasing in particular is a catch-all term: localities may be small geographical entities (such as electoral wards); small GP practice-based areas; larger geographical areas (such as old district health authorities within new larger health authorities); or larger GP-defined areas such as a catchment area for consortia of GP practices, whether fundholders, non-fundholders or both.

Initiatives such as the Nottingham non-fundholding consortium reflect a reaction against fundholding which seeks to combine improvement in provision with acceptable management costs. (To that extent, it is predictable that the Labour Party has latched onto the initiative as a vision for the future) (see, for example, *British Medical Journal* 1994, 309, 930–3). Such a large group of non-fundholders feeds into a medical advisory group (to which fundholders also contribute) and then into central health authority planning, rather than a locality-based model.

About half of the district health authorities in existence in 1995 had, on paper, a locality purchasing model within their district, although the variation in both nature and scope of this was great. Often different approaches apply within the same health authority, for different services. This raises another important point: GPs' involvement in such schemes often reflects specific needs for specific services and it would be dangerous to assume that any resulting model is a generic one suitable for comprehensive planning or comprehensive input into planning within a health authority.

A survey conducted within one large region (incidentally considered innovative in involving GPs) suggested that two-thirds of GPs did not consider themselves as having *any* involvement in long-term planning and of the third that did, 'long-term planning' consisted predominantly of 'practice development plans', practice visits and forum-type activities rather than more substantial 'planning with teeth'. It was also interesting to note that a minority of GPs wished personally to be involved in such activities but that more than 90% considered that GPs (presumably others!) should be involved (Harrison, 1996).

Naturally the means of involvement, whether at central health authority level or locally, can vary considerably, from election to (central) executive committees or local advisory groups, open meetings to strategy-based activities such as practice development plans. Perhaps predictably, the most important incentives for participation (in whatever) were seen as remuneration and secretarial support (Harrison, 1996).

It is important therefore to distinguish the type of input by GPs (ranging from the strategic to the purely operational) from the scale or salience of involvement and also from the means of involvement. It is too early to define the dominant trend for GP involvement and, again, it is worth keeping in mind the good old-fashioned concept of 'horses for courses'.

At the macro level, it is true that 'countries with more highly developed systems of primary care tend to have lower health care costs' (Starfield, 1994). The danger is that the cost-effective nature of primary care as gatekeeper can be undermined by elaborate schemes promoting GP-based planning which are not justified in terms of outcome and benefit. Combining the gatekeeping role with influence by GPs in changing behaviour by secondary providers and also the balance of care between primary and secondary may be achieved in certain 'group practice' health maintenance organisations in the USA. The challenge, then, is to seek any such advantages within a British context.

To return to some of the considerations at the beginning of this chapter, it is important to remind ourselves of the possible incompatibility of 'democracy' and 'technocracy'. Whether individual patients or citizens or general practitioners are consulted about desired services or not, their commissioning of services may reflect local wishes *or* (national or regional) research-based evidence on health gain. At the end of the day, there may be conflicts between utilitarianism and equality of access and between the role of the health service as responding to people's wishes (which may include rescue and care) and its role in sponsoring successful 'outcome'.

There is a clear tension, if not contradiction, between averaging utilities across individuals in order to construct quality adjusted life years (QALYs) and the like, and valuing individuals' choices. Individuals value outcomes differently. While resources are unlikely to permit every individual's choice of outcome, different means of consulting the public or general practitioners are likely to lead to different chosen outcomes.

It may be inevitable that different preferences are 'averaged out'. (That is, different individuals' utilities are compared, as economists would put it.) Nevertheless, when different value is put on different treatments for the same condition (at different costs, perhaps, as well), then ranking preferences to decide priorities is problematic. Unless clinicians are 'ordered' which treatment to prescribe, whether or not a condition is considered 'cost effective' to treat may well be indeterminate. (It depends how you do it, for whom.) Thus do rationing methodologies fall down. Paradoxically, local communities' preferences may best be served by letting GPs decide when or whether to refer them to services planned by regions involving both GPs and the public.

Finally, if priorities are to be made, this should involve planners (including epidemiologists), clinicians, economists and the public (in some variant). Needs and demands have to be reconciled with cost. If this does not produce national priorities, there will be the problem of denying NHS care to people as a result of their postcode or purchaser's choice.

Additionally, even national priorities should not mean other services are subject to 'blanket bans'. Clinicians may be able to demonstrate significant personal benefit, for individuals, from services judged inadequately cost effective on average. And as a result, providers can help to 'feed into' the debate about priorities and services. All this incidentally requires purchasers and providers to be co-operative or, indeed, partners in an integrated organisation.

6 The consequences revisited

INTRODUCTION

All countries in the world are facing difficult choices, both political and economic, as regards the financing and provision of health care. At root, these stem from the world economy in which revived capitalism demands low taxes and pruning of welfare states within nations. In particular, and most relevant to comparisons with Britain, the introduction of market mechanisms into broadly public health-care systems occurred (although in different forms) in countries in Scandinavia, in The Netherlands and strongly in New Zealand. These developments were based on a hope or faith that new systems could increase productivity at the very least. In many other countries also, similar trends and pressures apply, including 'developing' countries where (under pressure from multilateral agencies such as the World Bank) there is pressure both to diminish the scope of the public sector and to introduce quasi-commercial mechanisms into public health services.

Another major trend was the 'export' (whether appropriately or not) of ideas from Britain to the countries of the former communist block. For this and other reasons, it is all the more important that independent assessment of the NHS reforms is conducted and publicised and it is equally important that such assessment goes beyond the merely 'technical' (stressing productivity and quantitative outputs as a result of reform) to include the political and social context of reform. Otherwise, naive transplanting of models or, indeed, hasty rejection of otherwise valuable insights may continue.

COMPARATIVE HEALTH REFORMS

Some commentators have seen a convergence in systems which have traditionally been different. It is now claimed, for example, that (despite remaining differences) US and British health care contain similar trends (such as what Alain Enthoven (1995) now calls 'managed care – managed competition').

By this hybrid phrase, Enthoven refers to competition specifically between comprehensive care organisations, such as health maintenance organisations in the United States. Individual consumers or their firms tend to be the buyers of coverage in the US and the competing organisations are, to use the somewhat confusing British language, integrated purchasers and providers. Health maintenance organisations buy packages of care either from within their own organisation or from outside contractors. One can talk *either* about the individual consumer or firm being the purchaser and the HMO being the provider *or* about the consumer choosing the purchaser: there is an analogy between the health authority (or consortium of GP fundholders) in Britain and the purchasing arm of the HMO. It is to some extent therefore a question of language, although it is important to be clear about terms.

Managed competition, in its British variant, is by now familiar as competition by providers for contracts from public purchasers (rather than individual consumers or citizens). 'Managed care' in the broadest sense actually refers to the integration of care packages through a clinical planning process, involving protocols for care, and can exist with or without managed competition.

The market route, or consumerist route, to further reform is to allow citizens/consumers to choose their 'health plan', in the sense described by the Clinton Plan in the US in 1994, or in the sense of the Dutch reforms, whereby individuals enrol with their chosen insurance company or sick fund. These 'plans' compete for clients on the basis of quality, access etc. (but not price, as the finance is public. Only top-up payments by individual clients, for services above the prescribed, or core, services, would be on the basis of price competition between health plans). The health plans might be called purchasers, in a British context, but purchasers competing for citizen enrolment. They might therefore be consortia of GP fundholders, new-style health authorities or even insurance companies. In order to compete, they would market their relations with providers, in terms of the latter's quality, suitability and so forth. To ensure that competition provided the full range of services which were covered publicly, it would be 'managed competition', meaning regulation to prevent (for example) 'niche marketing' such that each plan specialised in different clinical services – resulting in what economists would call 'monopolistic competition' (many suppliers but with differentiated products of interest or use to different groups of consumers). For example, one plan might be geared to the needs of heart patients, another to eye patients and so on. This would lead to local monopolies.

Additionally, 'managed competition' would refer to regulation to ensure access by all, without 'cream skimming' to exclude sicker, poorer or otherwise more expensive clients. This would necessitate public resource allocation to health plans in proportion to the morbidity and age profiles of their members – a familiar concept in Britain, only now on the basis of chosen health plans rather than spatial health authorities.

This was the option considered by the government in 1993 (confidential interviews). The alternative route – to reintegration of the NHS – is to restore public planning (in as updated a form as possible, to allow some of the rigidities of the pre-reform NHS to be removed). Labour followed the latter route after 1997 in spirit, if not always in detail. Thus the choice was between more, and different, markets on the one hand and abandonment of markets on the other hand, in favour of population-based planning.

TYPES OF MARKET

Our own research reported in this book *confirms* the view that, even before the election of 1997, there was 'not really a market' in the NHS. There was a combination of central management under political direction and the use of market incentives in certain circumstances. It becomes a matter of theology whether this is described as 'managing the market' or simply managing and planning the service. An earlier evaluation of the NHS reforms (Robinson and Le Grand, 1994) drew upon a definition of the quasi-market in terms of replicating an actual market in a public sector context.

The assumption was that to meet certain allegedly agreed objectives for the National Health Service (efficiency, effectiveness by certain definitions, quality in certain senses, 'consumerism' and also equity), market mechanisms could be used. In terms of values or prescriptions, there seemed to be an assumption that the best means of meeting these objectives was through market mechanisms. That is, the ideological thrust of the NHS reforms (that planning (never really carefully defined) had failed) seemed to be accepted. In other words, in order to achieve *desiderata* for the NHS as well as for other public services (education, housing, social care), it was important to define the conditions for a successful market, such that the *desiderata* could be achieved.

These conditions were familiar:

- 'perfect competition' among providers (and possibly competition on the purchasing side);
- behaviour by providers as 'maximising' and self-interested institutions with, by implication rather than assertion, adequate cohesion and leadership within the organisation to achieve these objectives;

- perfect and symmetrical information (or, in practice, one might say adequate information 'on both sides');
- 'transactions costs' (costs associated with contracting rather than planning) which are under control or justified in terms of benefit;
- adequately low costs of entry to and possibility of exit from the market by providers;
- and various other definitions from economics. For example, long-term economies of scale would undermine the possibility of combining 'marginal cost pricing' and 'profit' or break-even. Marginal cost pricing is a tenet of welfare economics justified in terms of signalling and social welfare.

These major conditions listed are necessary rather than sufficient conditions for success of markets. In the technical sense, markets are neutral with regard to equity; meeting certain criteria of equity, in the NHS 'quasi-market', would require effective behaviour by purchasers – whether acting at the behest of government or higher tiers within the National Health Service or acting within regulated market conditions if purchasers are also seen as competitive entities with their own 'objective functions'.

In reviewing these conditions, our judgement as to actual events is as follows.

1. Market structures are inadequate to ensure competition. This emerges from our (and other) surveys. What is more, countervailing policy, such as rationalisation of services and mergers in pursuit of other objectives, diminishes the scope for appropriate market structures still further.

   After May 1997, the new Labour government identified the need for reconfiguration of the hospital sector, both to ensure appropriate quality and to save resources. 'Health action zones' are to provide civil input into this process (Dobson, 1997).
2. There is an area of 'fudge' when it comes to the behaviour of providers. That is, they are not 'self-interested' and are clearly not 'maximising' profit, surplus or any other bottom line. If one is to obey the laws of the market and obtain the public good from private vice, therefore, there is confusion of message to providers. Some are or were happy to be vicious; others are less so. The conflicting messages of competition and collaboration mean that neither the benefits of markets nor the benefits of planning are achieved. It is a familiar and true dictum that the problem with both markets and planning is that they deviate from textbook prescriptions. Indeed, in pure theory, the ideal market may achieve the results of the ideal planning system, just as the ideal planning system was designed in certain socialist economic theorists' prescriptions, earlier this century, to achieve the 'textbook' advantages of the market in terms of allocation.

Additionally, there are too many conflicting objectives within trusts, which undermine the achievement of overall or dominant behaviour patterns to ensure appropriate market behaviour. Clinical directors in clinical departments may undermine overall trust policy, if that is indeed adequately defined. (In practice, trusts lurch, punch-drunk, from one central directive to another, often fire-fighting the latest financial crisis en route.) Admissions policies in particular specialties; how to handle waiting lists and 'trade-offs' with other social obligations; how to 'trade off' clinical benefit, cost and reimbursement through the contracting mechanisms in operation: all these are grey areas which prevent adequately focused market behaviour.

3. Observations have already been made in Chapter 4 concerning asymmetries in information on power which allow purchasers and providers to 'play games' with each other.
4. It is always a million-dollar question as to whether the transactions costs of market mechanisms are either less than the costs of hierarchical organisation and/or less than the benefits of operating through market contracting. Given the absence of markets in other respects, it is very likely indeed that the transactions costs of 'playing at markets' are unjustified, given other features of the post-reform NHS at present.
5. Given economic barriers to entry into the marketplace, one aspect of government policy which may implicitly have been designed to 'sharpen up' the market was the policy of a 'primary care-led NHS'. This is at least in part (we assume from interviews and overall judgement) to be informed by the desire to 'sharpen up' the hospital sector and to provide alternative sources and locations of secondary services in order to allow greater competition. In practice, it is proving a crude device, in that the pressure on hospitals is not necessarily appearing at the right points (if, indeed, it were possible to define these).

So we return to the question raised in analysing the data and case studies: was the market an end or a means for the former Conservative administrations? Despite some ideological genuflections towards the former, it is clear it was generally the latter. A further question then arises: is it the best means of achieving increasingly tightly defined planning objectives? The creation of quasi-markets in the public sector extends well beyond the National Health Service. Indeed, at an earlier stage of the reforms, the model of the self-governing trust was derived from the model of the self-governing school in education.

Another means of characterising the appropriate form of market for the NHS was to describe an industrial market rather than a spot market or 'banana market'. That is, instead of competitive forces based on transparent prices and decentralised decision making, the 'market' in the NHS consists in long-term stable relationships between purchasers and providers. One industrial model sometimes suggested is that of the relationship between an airline and an aircraft manufacturer. Long-term guarantees as to the suitability of planes or engines, long-term contracting and symbiotic working between the two are the order of the day.

In the NHS, the signals were mixed. The above might be the logic of planning for longer term needs and also providing adequate self-management by the components of the service and in particular providers. Nevertheless, during the naive, early phase of the NHS reforms, we saw the hustle and bustle and indeed macho behaviour of public sector managers 'playing at' banana markets. Some 'first-wave' GP fundholders, for example, seemed to think of the market like this and the 'knock-on' effects of their behaviour were something that nascent purchasers were either unable or unwilling to consider. Analysis of Chapter 4 suggests that there is a dissonance between the longer term requirements of the service and the particular mode of operation of the 'short-termist' market.

When it comes to equity, it can again be argued that either a planning route or a market route is possible. If, for example GP fundholders are thought to indulge in 'cream skimming' (screening out patients with adverse financial consequences), then there are different means of handling this. Plans or regulations can be made. Alternatively, the resource allocation mechanism which allocates funds to fundholders can be rendered more sophisticated. Again, either is possible in theory. It is a question of which is most appropriate, in practice, in terms of cost and benefit. The costs of contracting with fundholders are high. Our own survey and case studies suggest that there is commonly an inverse relationship between fundholder income (small) and management resources spent on it (large).

Inequity may derive from variation in local purchasers' decisions. Treatment criteria may vary and therefore 'where one lives' can affect either what type of service is available or where one has to travel to get it. It can be observed that the NHS always varied widely for historical reasons rather than simply because of differences in need. Nevertheless, institutionalising differences through specific incentives may be a different matter. It is a question of how one works to provide a national service.

It has already been pointed out that fundholding may weaken a needs-based service on the basis of undermining long-term business planning by or for providers. Furthermore, given both institutional autonomy for providers and tight financial control (if not local 'profit maximisation'), there is a sharpened incentive for separate trusts to pass the buck to each other. That is, there is provider–provider buck passing, both from one acute trust to another and from acute to community trusts and vice versa. There can also be purchaser–purchaser buck passing, as fundholders seek to shift expensive care out of their own budgets. There is certainly purchaser–provider buck passing, as discussed in Chapter 3 in terms of purchasers 'expecting the earth' under the contract and expecting the public to blame the provider rather than the purchaser. There can also be provider–purchaser buck passing, as providers 'work to contract' more rigidly than in the pre-reform NHS. Our case studies produced significant confidential (and open) testimony to various forms of buck passing.

Perhaps the ultimate buck passing in the marketplace is from government to the NHS as a whole. In order to prevent debates about availability and comprehensiveness of health services occurring at the national level, it is convenient to the government that purchaser blames provider and provider blames purchaser. While the public still thinks in terms of overall funding, the long-term trend may be to deflect attention from wider public debates about financing, as the good old-fashioned policy of 'divide and rule' works in practice.

DEVOLUTION?

It was observed at the beginning of this book that a useful manner of characterising the change in the NHS after the reforms is to point not so much to a new purchaser/provider split as to the devolution of that split. Instead of an amalgam of regional and health authority planning (which, for example, reserves money for specialised services), the devolution of actual purchasing budgets (if not of real power in determining priorities) means that both the nature of service provision and the cost of organising that provision may be altered. Cost, in short, may be increased through increased transactions. The nature of the service may be altered, in some cases by design (as 'rationing' changes decisions) but also in some cases by accident. There is a 'problem of collective action' here potentially. Purchasing of specialised services may require intricate collaboration between different purchasers (including many fundholders when they hold the total budget for patient care). Organising this joint purchasing may be difficult.

There is an analogy with taxation. Even if one assumes adequate altruism to wish to pay taxes for social purposes, there is no point in paying tax if others do not do likewise and the yield is not enough to do something worthwhile. That is, voluntary tax may fail not only because of self-interest but for reasons of organisation and mobilisation. The same is sometimes the case with over-decentralised purchasing. Only organisation from above, reaction to crisis or a mixture of local good will and luck may produce the right result. There is evidence that the removal of regions and decentralisation of budgets for specialised services leads either to omissions or bureaucratic and often inflexible means of co-ordinating over-decentralised purchasing through service-specific consortia. For example, in one region, heart transplants were 'allocated' to districts (one or two each). Yet what happens if all the need fell in one or two districts (as it did)? This is but one example of how expecting consortia of districts to agree contracts for specialised services may create rigidity. It is indeed an issue affecting all contracting. If providers are funded only for supplying services if they are within specific contracts for specific purchasers, rigidity is built in. What at first might seem greater precision and strong planning/purchasing may in fact come to mean subjugation of clinical need to financial lottery.

Other areas in which devolution (again stressing contracting and organisation rather than broader political devolution) created particular problems in meeting objectives are manpower planning, including training; local pay; and private finance. Manpower planning and training are now left to trusts and consortia of trusts, with almost indecipherable arrangements for commissioning training and the dangers that longer term needs are unaddressed and that the system is costly yet inadequate.

Local pay and private finance are worth further comment, in that they have become significant planks of the new health service, although mentioned less at the launch of the reforms.

Whatever one thinks of the existence or otherwise of a market, it is important to trace the extent to which concern over the labour force has lain behind various reforms of the NHS. What became the Griffiths Inquiry recommending general management originally began as a reaction to the health service strikes of 1982, when Mrs Thatcher commissioned an enquiry into the cost of various cadres of NHS manpower. Roy Griffiths wished to broaden his terms of reference, rather than consider manpower as separate from broader management issues. The rest is history.

In 1988, after the announcement of the Prime Minister's Review of the National Health Service, the use of market mechanisms to allow providers to 'sub-contract' for labour more flexibly and reduce the power of labour was an overt agenda, as proclaimed at the time by David Willetts (now an MP, then Director of the Centre for Policy Studies and formerly the member of Mrs Thatcher's Policy Unit with responsibility for health) (Willetts, 1988).

Much has now been written on local pay and related issues, including demand for and supply of different cadres of the NHS labour force. Alongside questions of pay are issues of reorganisation of the labour force, the so-called 're-profiling' which some see as a search for greater efficiency and flexibility and others see as a search for intensified labour and exploitation.

Concerning the Private Finance Initiative, our case study interviews revealed that it is a source of major frustration. Again, it is the stasis caused by a combination of central bureaucracy and mandatory 'local initiative', in the search for private finance, which seems to be at the heart of the frustration. There is both an ideological and a practical debate about the merits or otherwise of seeking private finance. In practice, it is proving to be a source of delay in capital development. The Labour government's attempt to streamline the PFI after May 1997 was a pragmatic reaction to the absence of public investment.

The PFI of course interfered with the market in that, in order to interest profit-taking companies in developments in the NHS, the contracting mechanisms of the market have to be suspended. Purchasers have to guarantee long-term support for local providers (sometimes ten years, in some cases much longer), under the tutelage of the region and possibly the national government. Otherwise the private investment would be considered too risky. Thus, the search for private finance takes precedence over the functioning of the market. As the first edition of this book pointed out (in Chapter 5), capital allocations are in essence central to planning. Whoever allocates capital is the planner, overtly or not. Private capital – and government decisions as to who gets it – is therefore another source of centralism in planning, despite the rhetoric.

As with the market itself, of course, the private finance policy was an initiative across the whole public sector and there is arguably evidence that it is less suited to the NHS than other sectors of the economy. In the NHS, the business of contracting for population needs may be distorted when providers have to seek specific 'profitable' business in order to service payback on private finance arrangements. Furthermore, the policy is an extremely expensive one for the public purse in the long run and may well not be justified in terms of benefit.

Perhaps the long-term effect of the NHS reforms, if not amended or changed substantially, was to enable such privatisation through the creation of institutions (such as quasi-autonomous and commercial provider trusts) which allow a gradual metamorphosis of the NHS into a mixed health-care economy.

SPECIFIC CONCLUSIONS

1. Funding

The NHS reforms were a reaction to a perceived problem of underfunding. At the level of political rhetoric, it was argued that efficiency improvements 'on the supply side' would remove or diminish this problem. This has not occurred.

2. The market as pressure

The creation of provider markets yet monopsonistic (single payer) funding could be said to create a structure whereby the 'market' consists in 'squeeze' on providers. Pluralism in purchasing as well as in provision might be considered to create a more balanced market. The GP fundholding policy has incorporated diversity in financing but, given the squeeze on finance, especially for the hospital sector, providers generally have to assemble a coalition of purchasers, around a dominant local health authority purchaser. This prevents a diversity in financing from becoming either a pluralism in financing or a full 'purchaser market'.

3. Remote purchasers

The purchaser is not the agent of the consumer (a tenet of normative welfare economics being that the consumer is the best judge of his own welfare and that interpersonal comparisons of utility are suspect) but is instead a conduit for a series of government policy initiatives. A survey of 40 health authorities (in the questionnaire reported in Chapter 5) suggested that only two of the 40 differed from the view that public consultation was primarily designed to legitimise actions which were intended in any case.

4. Original motivation

Different intentions, at the time of the NHS reforms, can be grouped as belonging to free-market liberals and right-wing Conservatives. Right-wing politicians tended to see the NHS internal market as a compromise in lieu of more thoroughgoing privatisation of provision, finance or both. Others believed that genuine public sector markets might emerge. Alain Enthoven's original recommendation (Enthoven, 1985) was for direct reimbursement of patient flows rather than leaving it to a formula, which he considered created rigidity. It was only later that the concept of self-governing trusts emerged (*Working for Patients*, Working Paper 1) and later still, that the concept of the purchaser/provider split emerged. Consumer choice of integrated health plan was the normative model which Enthoven had in mind, however, even in 1984–85 (based on the US health maintenance organisation). His recommendations in the US were for consumer choice health plans, based on the replacement of the dominant third-party payment, fee-for-service system with a system of competing health maintenance organisations for which all citizens would be eligible in varying degrees.

This continuing normative influence has created a tension in Britain: a desire for further separation between the purchaser and the provider yet an awareness that the most effective health maintenance organisations in the United States benefit from integration between the administrative entity purchasing health care and providers. More thoroughgoing marketeers and those on the Right seeking more radical reform tend to stress a greater role for private financing and also for greater consumer choice within the public sector. Before the 1997 election there was a tension on the Left between those who wish to utilise fully the purchaser/provider split and those who saw it as a disruption to an integrated NHS. Often, of course, such differences are more in presentation rather than detailed policy. A desire to be seen to be 'forward looking' or wary of further organisational change produces soundbites more favourable to the purchaser/provider split. There is a tension between 'radicalism' in the sense of restoring a public integrated NHS ('old radicalism') and 'modernisation' in the sense of accepting the reforms as the basis of future change.

In consequence, the purchaser/provider split in the context of global purchasing health authorities is often seen as the compromise solution but this is at the level of political compromise rather than as a result of research showing it achieves objectives in a cost-effective manner.

5. Are the reforms distinct?

What are now known as the 'NHS reforms' were all things to all men. To those who specifically favoured the reforms, there was a tendency to see problems within the system as related to the remnants of the old system; to those who opposed the reforms, there was a tendency to see perverse incentives and awkward consequences as the result of the reforms themselves. The reform process embraced not only the policy for a market and the policy for a purchaser/provider split, but a whole raft of other central initiatives. The task of rendering these initiatives compatible has downplayed markets in themselves and it would be fair to categorise the NHS reform process as a generic management reform. The absence of markets has led to the advertising of contestability rather than competition in the supply of services to purchasers. Naturally, the contracting system allows the possibility of contestability but one is in a murky area when one seeks to distinguish between planning choices (always available to health authorities in the old system, whether properly used or not) and the so-called 'contestability' of the market system.

6. Collaboration

The fact that the average trust still derives much of its income from the local health authority puts the above comments into perspective. Indeed, it is perhaps in 'competition' between acute and primary or community care that tensions were fomented quite deliberately, to seek to stimulate alternative modes of provision in the hope that these are either more cost effective or perhaps simply cheaper. Here choices had to be made. Although national policy in 1995 (conducted through regions) seemed to be to encourage competition between acute and community trusts, there was later a greater thrust towards 'collaboration', whether this is organised contractually (through a 'lead provider' model whereby one type of trust subcontracts for services to another, for patient groups) or through patient-oriented protocols which seek to regulate relations between different types of trusts (for patients requiring pre-hospital and after-hospital care).

In the light of data concerning reliance of a trust on a single purchaser and also the fact that most health authorities' funds are allocated to only three or four key providers, the relationship between 'purchasers' and 'providers' may well be similar to that existing before the reforms. Purchasers are seeking to ensure comprehensive health care for their resident population and require close relationships with local providers. Whether one conceptualises providers as local monopolies, in market language, or simply as local public services is a matter of theology to some extent, although providers' self-perceptions will affect their behaviour.

In other words, is selling their product more important than local loyalty? As the Sheffield case study shows, one provider's behaviour in this respect can have knock-on effects for others. Whatever the motivation of the provider or of its key actors (especially board members and clinical directors), the requirement to break even annually means that aggressive behaviour by another local provider may create at the very least defensive behaviour and 'niche marketing' by the affected provider.

One generalisation from our research is that, in the initial years of the reforms, providers often sought development of 'new products' in order to extend their markets. Later they have tended to return to responding to their host purchasers' plans. Ironically innovation is probably stimulated more through a close working relationship between purchaser and provider than through the purchaser viewing itself purely as a 'market regulator', which is sometimes the image for the new health authorities with the rise of fundholding.

7. Mutual dependency

Where the host health authority purchaser is less dominant as funder (and incidentally this is most likely where there are large numbers of GP fundholders), GP fundholders often operated on the providers' behalf to sway the health authority's purchasing agenda towards a common goal. That is, they not only use their own purchasing power to influence the provider but also use both formal and informal methods to influence the health authority.

The fact that health authorities are swayed by such action is a result not so much of relative market power but of their appreciation that GPs as health-care providers are a valuable source of information and expertise. This is an example of how purchasers must use information from providers. Short of national and regional information being available for local use, local purchaser–provider symbiosis is perhaps inevitable. Health authorities will also seek to incorporate non-fundholding GPs into such planning exercises. Another reason why health authorities must 'bring GPs, especially fundholders, on board' is that unco-ordinated purchasing can have unforeseen or undesirable effects upon providers. Survival is the latter's imperative, at a time when static income and rising capital charges as well as 'efficiency squeeze' are putting significant pressure upon trusts.

8. Bureaucratic costs

It is impossible accurately to compare data on costs for particular activities pre- and post-reform in the NHS and certainly to attribute exact changes to particular elements of the reforms such as the market, purchaser/provider split and the like. Nevertheless, it is possible to trace examples of high bureaucratic and transactions costs and to seek to reduce these without affecting output or outcomes significantly. It could of course be argued that such costs are an inevitable transitional burden, if new arrangements with associated benefits are to be achieved. Whether or not this is the case, there is significant scope (for example) for costs associated with fundholding to be diminished, through longer term contracting, larger scale purchasing and, arguably, through a lean but effective input by GPs into the purchasing/planning process rather than the continuation of fundholding.

Equally, there is evidence that a fully institutionalised purchaser/provider split replicates costs and functions at both provider and purchaser level which are necessary only for the administration of short-term contracting rather than for more strategic purposes. With this in mind, our recommendation is that the purchaser/provider *distinction* is considered as just that, rather than as a market-oriented *split*. Robust management within providers should not mean that they are not part of the local health service. Indeed, considering the origin of the reforms as a means for directly financing patient flows and workload, it is the (relatively small) increment of flows from one health authority to another which makes it important as to which institution, the health authority or the recipient providers, is financed for such.

It is interesting to note that this is one of the areas which has troubled the Labour Party; it is against the purchaser/provider split in a general ideological sense (or at least was until very recently) but accepts that, if providers are to be funded in relation to workload, they may need to receive the finance directly. This makes them a separate administrative entity from the purchaser.

The only way to get around this is either to abolish local purchasing and replace it with regional planning or to channel finance through the recipient health authority for translation to its 'directly managed provider'; or for providers to receive income directly for flows, yet be politically accountable to the local health authority.

All of these options have advantages and disadvantages. Regional planning sounds remote and bureaucratic but may actually be less costly. If the region comes to mirror the Swedish County Council, it may be the most appropriate organ for 'democratic' input into planning and commissioning. On the other hand, holding providers accountable to much more local purchasers (which is the thinking behind 'locality purchasing' below the level of the health authority), in order to ensure that local populations needs are met, necessitates some form of local contracting. Again, it is a question of costs and benefits. Having self-managing providers yet local accountability (to provider boards representing the locality) may itself be a politically attractive solution – and seemed originally to be the solution proposed by the Labour Party in its document *Renewing the NHS* (1995). It may, however, be cumbersome in practice. Local provider authorities may be politically dominated (in the negative sense of that term) and interfere with 'good management' and, additionally, their relationship with purchasing authorities will be unclear. Again, if the providers are not market entities, then what do the boards actually do?

This way of thinking leads one to a solution whereby providers have their management boards but are neither separate authorities nor have non-executive members. One is back in the realm of the 'unit' which existed prior to the NHS reforms but after the Griffiths Inquiry's recommendations were implemented!

9. Management complexity

Although most providers have one (or two) dominant purchasers, the fact that they have to market themselves to a variety of purchasers (including fundholders) means that different purchasers will have different requirements. Different maximum waiting times for outpatients is one example.

To quote one case study (a director of service development):

> I have seen this in Birmingham ... I have seen it where the GPs actually select which patients come into the hospital themselves and the bureaucracy at the hospital end in trying to manage that is incredible. At some point the system would fall apart because in theory what would happen is, you will send GPs a list of patients; they will tell you who they want to come in; the number of patients that they want to come in is beyond the capacity that you can fit in; and it does not leave you anywhere to put the urgent patient ... That is an extreme view but I think that is what is going to happen and you could have fifty contracts in theory all of which specify different access times. It is crackers, the management involved in that; it is unbelievable.

The interviewer's next question suggested that the hospital could take a firm stance and say there is only so much variety to be tolerated. This produced the reply, 'Well, that is all right, but then you get a trust down the road, a bit of a maverick, which is prepared to do that for whatever reason: things will catch up with him later but for now they are prepared to do it'.

In other words, 'short-termism' in the market can be a negative-sum game: all lose or the result is a net loss!

10. Fundholding: a metamorphosis

The way in which hospitals deal with fundholders varies and is dependent upon a number of factors. Changes in calculations for their budgets as fundholding becomes more salient ('both wider and deeper', as there are more fundholders with budgets for more care) may lead to less differential advantage for fundholders. In our study, some fundholders' patients were disfavoured rather than favoured, often at the request of financially stretched fundholders.

At one extreme, fundholding can be generalised such that consortia of fundholders become *de facto* the new health authorities, although often justified as more locally based purchasing. There was initially a mismatch in policy between the fundholding scheme being voluntary and regions and health authorities being set targets for the achievement of more fundholding. That is, it was voluntary at the practice level and mandatory at the authority/regional level.

It might be argued that, even if fundholders' patients have differential advantage in terms of waiting times, if waiting times improve for all, then there are no absolute losers. (A strict egalitarian could nevertheless still object to this.) Of course, improved waiting times may simply reflect 'waiting time initiatives' rather than the institutions of either fundholding or the market in general.

One particular study carried out as part of the Keele MBA programme studied three hospitals over five years of the fundholding scheme and discovered that in one of the three, a certain and significant bias existed in favour of non-fundholding practices in terms of waiting times (Ambler, 1996). Again, Labour's approach to fundholding, in office, is geared to 'getting the best of both worlds'. It is hoped that prohibiting separate waiting lists for fundholders' patients and the rest will restore equity. But retaining the paraphernalia while regulating it tightly may be very cumbersome and will not solve the problems of administrative cost, on the one hand, and the countervailing need for higher tier planning, on the other.

11. Overall management costs

Overall management costs have risen significantly since 1989. The bulk of these costs has appeared in trusts, with up to 10% of their costs being management. This is not a 'criticism' of trusts, in that the dynamics of the system necessitate this. An overall conclusion, however, is that the transactions costs (and most of the additional costs) are connected with the contracting process – annual marketing; annual contracting; annual monitoring and related activities. Moderately greater investment in higher tiers could release (not vast but moderate) sums currently 'tied up' with management costs. Some precision in contracting might be lost. But targeting high administrative cost is important.

We have not researched the operation of capital charging. Currently, however, the policy seems to act as a disincentive to appropriate investment (because new capital is expensive yet current prices are being cut) and also as an incentive to asset stripping in that reduction of capital charges has become a financial necessity at a time of increasing squeeze. Since a real market is not operating, the policy is in effect conducted through purchasers. Purchasers allocate the costs of capital to providers as part of the purchasing package and it operates as a bureaucratic exercise rather than as an incentive to significant innovation via providers. It is also responsible for increasing management costs.

12. Failure in basic objectives

A major conclusion, as already stated in Chapter 3, is that the money does not follow the patient. Coupled with the 'cost equals price rule' plus efficiency savings in a context whereby hospitals are not allowed to use surpluses to increase capital or resources, a trust which takes on more patients may end up having to cut prices to such a point that clinical quality is seriously threatened. This is a severe 'efficiency trap'. Neither major objective of the reforms – rewarding efficiency and letting flows of patients occur more easily – has been achieved.

GENERAL CONCLUSION

Research for this book has suggested that the 'NHS reforms' in the sense of the market and purchaser/provider split were in fact the latest in a long line of management reforms to the NHS. After the foundation of the NHS in 1948, the first major structural reorganisation occurred in 1974. On paper, the 1991 reforms were the antithesis of the 1974 reforms, which instituted tiers (districts, areas and regions) which came to be perceived as a bureaucratic, top-heavy 'planning' reorganisation. Although the management structures created by the 1974 reforms led to what became known as consensus management and allowed the representation of different interests both in management teams and on health authorities, there was some consensus by the early 1980s that a leaner and more flexible organisation was required. To some extent, this perception parallelled the rise and fall of 'grand planning' in both public and private sectors more generally.

Nevertheless, the market was more metaphor than reality, in the 1991 NHS reforms. Ironically, these reforms also created a significant quantity of bureaucracy and allowed the representation of a whole range of (very different) interests within the National Health Service.

What remains, in a long line of continuity, is the tension between central policy making and local initiative, with the balance shifted further to the former despite rhetoric suggesting the opposite. Increasingly the costs of market mechanisms, or rather the procedures which go under the name of market mechanisms, are being recognised, although it is politically difficult for the Conservatives to disown major elements of their own reforms, and also politically difficult for Labour in government to suggest another reorganisation (smacking of 'turning the clock back').

The creation of the purchaser/provider split creates the potential for privatisation of and within provision and the Private Finance Initiative could well represent the first substantial privatisation (both of capital supply and of ownership). The purchaser/provider split has been interpreted by some commentators as merely a technical device within a fully public health-care system. If the reforms are to be more than the latest 'structural fix', however, it is via this opening to greater private involvement and greater public/private symbiosis in provision. Coupled with limitations on finance and public purchasing, a more pluralistic system on the demand side as well as on the supply side may develop, under certain economic and political assumptions. If this is so, it can fairly be said that the institutions of the reforms have rendered this approach more structurally possible as well as rendering such a development more seemingly inevitable.

The co-ordinating of 'purchasing' is of course an important objective and the reforms may have 'sharpened the mind wonderfully' as regards (what would previously have been called) planning. Most health-care systems face the challenge of allocating resources appropriately to purchasers (in many ways, the Clinton reform in the US sought indirectly to do this). The danger in Britain is that we fragment this process just as a variety of countries are seeking to do the opposite – to create larger insurers/purchasers capable of greater equity and more strategic planning.

Irrespective of levels of financing for the National Health Service, the two main alternative scenarios for the future are a replacement of or (more likely politically) 'tidying up' of the reforms and a diminution of the costs associated with 'feeding the beast' and administering the new system, on the one hand, and an undermining of an integrated National Health System as we have known it, on the other. Since political choices will in part determine which option is taken, whether the reforms are interpreted by historians as revolutionary, evolutionary or a blind alley remains to be seen.

At the broader level, there is a danger that Britain will become locked in a downward spiral in public health care. The political pressure for tax cuts leads not only to cutting public expenditure in the short term, but selling off assets which create longer term needs to cut expenditure (since short-term expenditure is only sustainable in part through the proceeds of such sales). This has been the story of the 1980s and early 1990s. While the NHS has so far escaped cuts, although it has failed to grow much, this will not remain true for long in the above scenario. (A cycle of decline means lower wages and worse conditions for the NHS's poorest employees, ironically with health consequences.)

Pressure on the public purse usually means pressure for private spending. We are seeking this in investment (the Private Finance Initiative) and in consumption/revenue expenditure (the growing acceptance of the 'fact' that a universal NHS is no longer affordable). As well as more predictable statements in 1995 from the political Right and from the former chairman of the NHS Trust Federation that the NHS will or must become a 'rump' service, we have seen commissions such as Healthcare 2000 (chaired by Sir Duncan Nichol yet including some commentors conventionally viewed as left of centre, such as Patricia Hewitt) arguing a similar case. Furthermore, expectations of the public sector are increasing, as government policy deliberately creates this alongside a more consumerist culture in any case and the more generously funded GP fundholding schemes may suggest (wrongly) that such a level of service is sustainable more generally. Disappointed expectations will help to undermine the public health service.

The so-called 'moral panic' may lead to sharper debates about rationing and whether it should be by service (QALY-type schemes) or by ability to pay. The reforms themselves were supposed to 'square the circle' of inadequate resources by increasing efficiency. The absence of any real evidence that they have done so, at the 'macro' level, will also help to create a sense of fatalism about 'what is affordable'.

There may be a vicious circle in financing the NHS. As incomes become more unequal, more progressive taxation would be necessary to maintain universal public services. Yet incomes are becoming more unequal as part of a political trend which includes lower, and more regressive, taxes. As a result, private affluence for some goes hand in hand with declining public services, including the NHS.

The question is, who and how many are the affluent 'some'? They may be the 'contented majority' – at least a majority of those who vote (which excludes the poor disproportionately, of course). Or, as the world economy employs cheaper labour sector by sector, even the previously secure may slip into lower incomes and/or insecurity. It may, over time, be less a case of the contented majority than of the contented minority. The difference (say, from the 1960s) is that the insecure majority no longer have redistribution within an affluent society as the solution, as economic power and capital move from the traditional Western countries to the sunrise and tiger economies, as well as new markets altogether. Imports from developing countries, often produced with outsourced capital from the West, are destroying jobs and communities in the West. This has not been lost on commentators from the Right (Goldsmith, 1994) as well as the Left.

Another question is, how much does 'public squalor' affect even the better off? (Traditional economic indicators of well-being are too narrow.) Crime, dirty streets, unsafe underground trains: these are sources of disquiet. As regards the NHS, it may at first seem that the better off are better off if they pay or insure themselves privately. Then they do not have to pay for others (i.e. for universal public services) through redistributive taxation.

But if it is more expensive so to do, they may be worse off than when they were paying for others through (limited) redistribution. If this is so, then the decline of the NHS would hit those who, on first inspection, do not need it. In such a scenario, it is shortsighted to say, 'We cannot afford the welfare state any more'; rather, 'We cannot afford not to have it'.

Of course, if new private financing and provision can be arranged economically, through using the inheritance of the NHS for those who can afford it, then a more inegalitarian and 'privatised' society is sustainable and 'rational' for the better off. At the end of the day, the question is an empirical one, although of course moral judgements can also be passed.

Tentative evidence and judgement would suggest that all have an interest in a reasonably comprehensive NHS, although 'extras' such as quicker treatment may be purchased by the better off without the need to pay publicly to ensure an economical service. When it comes to 'heavy duty' and emergency care, however, public suits all.

Individuals may feel these services too can be purchased privately. But building up a private network is expensive, compared to the inheritance available through the NHS. An analogy exists with purchasers, after the NHS reforms, seeking cheap deals at 'marginal cost'. In the long run, though, these may undercut the very providers who can presently provide them, unless the longer term investment is also furnished. Before this is done, services may have collapsed or been lost. Whether we are talking about private purchasers or NHS purchasers, money has to be spent recreating the network after (unintended) losses and gaps.

In today's NHS, we see the potential beginnings of this process and currently that is one of the reasons why planning is being resurrected by the 'back door', as central government (the Department of Health) and regional offices work directly with providers (hospitals, in the main) to preserve a viable service. Leave it to 'purchasers' and unintended consequences would ensue. Local purchasing may close (needed) local services, by default rather than by design. In practice, local purchasing (by GP fundholders, localities or whatever) will simply be a case of choosing from an already typed menu in an already chosen restaurant. It is who opens and closes the restaurants and plans the menus that matters. The rest is just transactions costs. GP fundholders, for example, who treasure their freedoms do not realise that they neither open the restaurant nor even type the menu. They merely purchase in an administratively expensive manner.

THE CENTRAL EFFECTS OF THE NHS REFORMS

The effects of the reforms range from the technical to the behavioural. That is, as well as consequences (for example) such as higher costs associated with certain contracting processes, there are changes such as the replacement of a culture based upon trust and co-operation with a new culture, which is an amalgam of contracts in the marketplace (instead of co-operative agreements) and top-down directives and controls. The implication is that human behaviour is economically determined, self-interested and yet responsive to the stick as well as the carrot. For, although the market reformers characterise the old NHS as based on 'command and control', it is the new NHS which has really seen central diktat. As Simon Jenkins put it, Margaret Thatcher 'completed what Bevan began: the nationalisation of the health service'. While Bevan's falling bedpans were intended to be heard at Westminster, Thatcher's were 'picked up, emptied, cleaned, counted and given a numbered place on the Whitehall shelf' (Jenkins, 1995).

It is in the interplay of the technical and the behavioural that the effects of the reforms can best be gauged and yet this interplay has not been evaluated so far (understandably, in that it is a difficult and not purely empirical task).

An illustration helps. Before the reforms, the funding of services in the NHS was a mixture of prospective and retrospective. The planning process (at least in theory) identified needs, and providers were funded after assumptions or models had been made about flows of patients, appropriate locations for hospitals and the like. This was the prospective bit. Where flows of patients (or workload for hospitals and other providers) were different from that anticipated, however, there was a mechanism for reimbursing the affected health authorities (which were of course in those days responsible for the providers). This mechanism was indirect (as it affected authorities' targets for future years rather than immediate finance) and imprecise (as the affected providers did not necessarily get the money).

This was the origin of the belief that, in the old NHS, 'extra workload was not rewarded' and that the money did not follow the patient. The reforms originated as a financial strategy.

What happened, however, was that a cultural (or ideological) solution was offered to a technical problem. It was not the 'old' culture that caused financial rigidity, although some argued that the old informal processes reinforced clinical power (in our view, a rather overstated case – effective management was capable of mobilising the organisation. And where it was not, it was unlikely that translating management desires into contracts was likely to help much). Rather, it was the divorce of planning (translated into capital allocations) and resource procedures (principally concerned with running costs) which was the problem.

This is the sense in which the reforms were a sledgehammer to crack a nut. In order to seek to ensure that providers were paid exactly for what they did, they were separated from health authorities (now to be purchasers); financed through contracts (which would supposedly measure their workload); and allegedly given incentives to do more in order to earn more.

Unfortunately, the problem inherent in the old NHS remained – the reforms were based on a faulty diagnosis compounded by a homeopathic cure which injected more of the problem. Unless every referral and admission were simply to be reimbursed retrospectively (the absence of adequate finance for which had led to the supposed problem in the first place), contracts would be prospective. They would thus be based not upon actual workload but upon estimated, planned or hypothesised workload.

At this point, what is more, the technical was compounded by the cultural. Politically, it could not be admitted that contracts would be financially inadequate to cover clinically sanctioned admissions or care. Theoretical acknowledgement of, and pieties about, rationing were one thing; denying a comprehensive NHS in practice was another (as Mr Dorrell's 1996 White Paper, *A Service with Ambitions*, again reinforced).

As a result, the market was hailed as the imminent source of increased productivity to such an extent that rationing would not be necessary. In 1992, Duncan Nichol, chief executive of the NHS, made this claim (although no doubt as the mouthpiece of ministers, especially given his later doubts as to the adequacy of prevailing finance for a comprehensive and universal service) (Nichol *et al.*, 1995).

In practice, this meant that purchaser was to be pitted against provider, to seek to squeeze more services out of block contracts. In public, ministers looked forward to the day when contracts would be precise, to when block contracts would be replaced by precise cost and volume, and even cost-per-case contracts. This would, however, wholly expose 'underfunding' (that is, the inadequacy of existing budgets for a comprehensive and universal service). The tongue that called for detailed contracting was therefore forked (even before the high costs of detailed contracting had become a political hot potato) because such detail would be highly inconvenient to ministers. Difficult decisions should be devolved, went the political maxim, not ladled onto a central plate.

More useful, therefore, were pricing rules for the market which assumed year-on-year efficiency savings and which did not reward increasingly productive (or cheap) providers, but did the opposite – built in their greater workload to future projections and financial targets without extra money. Lower costs, or 'efficiency', meant lower prices, by central diktat.

Thus the 'efficiency trap' of the old NHS was magnified. And to add to this, the new purchaser/provider split had the following effects.

- It led to high management costs, through contracting, especially where GP fundholding was relevant (with the costs of fundholding estimated to double management costs).
- It led to a bias towards a 'banana market', in the early days of the reforms, with purchasers having a naive expectation that they could shop around as if from a market stall.
- It led to perverse incentives, including cost shifting, inappropriate

performance and outcome measures (in order to 'measure something' and market it) and the possibility of adverse selection. Patients with high costs and low political visibility would be even less attractive than under the old system, unless 'strong purchasing existed.' Our research, as well as others', suggests that purchasers are far too squeezed financially to do much more than respond to governmental directives and meet existing demand as far as possible.

- It allowed providers to market their wares to the public and to GPs, constraining health authorities and planners when they sought to meet unfashionable needs. This was the opposite of the justification for the purchaser/provider split, based as it was on the idea that purchasers could focus on needs without the bother of being responsible for providers. But an absence of responsibility had a downside – it allowed providers to go over their heads and appeal to the 'contented majority' (Galbraith, 1992) with fashionable new services for the relatively better off. This has probably been compounded by fundholding, if the president of the Association of GP Fundholders is right to state that fundholders would go private rather than lose fundholding status (a repeated threat from Rhidian Morris, the president of the Association of GP Fundholders, in 1995 and 1996). They could only do so if their clients/patients were the better off, on aggregate.
- It prevented an integrated organisation from agreeing its objectives and seeking to meet these on the basis of trust and the ethos of public service. In particular, accountability was now narrowly defined in terms of financial accountability of providers to purchasers. A local provider, for example, is no longer part of an integrated organisation which is 'of the community'. Before the reforms, patients from outside the authority (locality) would admittedly not have a 'purchaser' allegedly representing their interests. But it was taken for granted that health authorities treated patients as referred, despite practical difficulties and funding problems. There was simply no need, given the public service ethos, to assume the need for financial accountability. Now, providers are financially accountable to a number of purchasers, but wider accountability is often lost.
- And, perhaps most importantly of all, it devolved planning (now demoted to commissioning and purchasing) to too low a level. Specialised services, the rationalisation of services generally, economies of scale: all these were threatened. Local providers, now autonomous trusts, sought market niches irrespective of long-term viability. Local purchasers, increasingly fundholders, took the worm's eye view.

It is difficult, as already stated, to disentangle the technical from the cultural and behavioural effects. But the above portrait may help in suggesting how policy and institutional changes provide a catalyst for behavioural change (on the part of managers and professionals in the NHS) in line with the 'New Right' ideology of the policy-makers.

THE REFORMS – AN UNORTHODOX VIEW

Since the 'reform' process began in the NHS with the Prime Minister's Review in 1988, the NHS has undergone a maelstrom of change. This is partly because a culture of change (often for change's sake) has taken over, but is also partly because the unintended consequences of the reform process require perpetual ironing out. The introduction of the market has created a see-saw between freeing up market forces and regulating the consequences of the market. Decentralised purchasing (fundholding) and regional planning to achieve economies of scale and appropriate siting of services have to be reconciled. And the 1996 'reorganisation' is the latest attempt to diminish bureaucracy by creating more.

Some people characterise the essence of the NHS reforms as the creation of a purchaser/provider split. This is partly true, but ignores the fact that purchasing *per se* is also a creation of the reforms. Purchasing/commissioning replaces the right of free referral by GPs and is an acknowledgement that not everything can be funded. Of course, there is also an opportunity then to involve populations (whether citizens or users) in deciding what is to be purchased but it nevertheless is (at heart) a means of legitimising a policy whereby the NHS is no longer to be a comprehensive service.

It is also a form of buck passing. The government passes the buck down the chain to purchasers. If, for example, palliative care for cancer sufferers is not to be made available (as recently highlighted in Bristol), then it is not the government which is superficially to blame but the local purchaser. The provider blames the purchaser for not funding the service; the purchaser argues that it must take responsibility for making choices or, more likely, that it is provider inefficiency or failure to make the money go around which is preventing more services being funded. Thus, buck passing from government to purchasers and on to providers is the norm of the new system. Tied in with this is the useful imperial policy of 'divide and rule', whereby the squabbling between purchasers and providers obscures the wider debate about desired levels of funding of the NHS, a debate which we can witness in The Netherlands and Sweden but not in the UK at present.

Of course, purchasers make choices, but they make these choices in constrained circumstances. Man makes his own history but not in circumstances of his choosing. It may be that where purchasing/commissioning is weak, the provider in effect determines which services will be 'purchased', as a result of either demonstrating strength *vis-à-vis* the purchaser (for market or advocacy reasons) or simply as a result of greater expertise. It is still, of course, the case that, in a system of 'overt purchasing' and a purchaser/provider split, even provider-led contracts will also make prioritisation or rationing characteristic of the system. For the purchaser still has to draw the line between funded and unfunded services – or people. However, it is useful to the government that this is seen as a characteristic of the system, rather than as a consequence of political and fiscal choices.

If one assumes a static budget for health care and growing expenditure on management costs involved with running the new (supposedly 'free') system, then it stands to reason that there is less money for patient care. This can only be justified if the dynamics of the new system, including the sophisticated choices made by the wonderful new managers and management systems, produce what economists would call more allocative efficiency or more technical efficiency or both. Allocative efficiency concerns 'doing better things' (to increase welfare, by economists' definitions); technical efficiency concerns producing more bang for the buck once one has decided what to do. Only if the total quantum of allocative and technical efficiency exceeds the additional costs of the new market system can it be justified, even in this basic technical way. And even if allocative efficiency gains dominate, the quantity of patient care may be cut below a politically acceptable level.

The 'opportunity cost' of spending more money on management (as a result of the reforms) is (less money on) patient care. Only if the new system produces gains greater than this loss could it be justified. And indeed the new system incurs new losses, as a fragmented NHS affects patient care. A further complication is that technical efficiency may simply be exploitation. If you halve the cost of labour and produce the same product, that may come out in a silly statistical or performance-managed system, as a near doubling of efficiency. But it is nothing to do with system improvement; it is simply increased intensification of labour. If one observes the wider social costs of such a system, a very different answer may be produced. As in debates about re-engineering of hospitals and reprofiling of workforces, it is important to attempt (difficult as it is) to separate out genuine efficiency factors and exploitation factors.

The government, by 1995, was panicking about the management costs of the new system. Crude directives to health authorities and trusts about cutting management costs to agreed percentages and totals reflect this panic. It is of course a hypocrisy. A system, the internal market, is created which has unforeseen management costs and bureaucratic spin-offs. The government's response is to preserve the system yet put increasing pressure on fewer managers in response to public disquiet. And often the 'management cuts' are not made in the most appropriate places, as the most powerful in organisations survive whether or not they are the most productive. High salaries in the NHS may be less than in the private sector, but they represent an escalation of costs, and inequity, unrelated to 'output' or improvements.

Most worrying of all is the capacity for further bureaucratic growth, as the various sorcerers' apprentices around the NHS create processes which soon run out of control. The purchaser/provider split itself means significant bureaucracy, as marketing, contracting, monitoring (and then going through the whole process all over again) take up valuable management resources. When it comes to consulting the public (supposedly a wonderful new panacea within the new system), we find both purchasers and providers doing it and, for example, voluntary groups having to deal with both, with roles and relationships neither clear nor demarcated.

Another aspect of the purchaser/provider split which causes problems is the incentive for the purchaser to 'hold back' money, on grounds of financial caution. Both fundholders and health authorities do this so, often, the appropriate workload is not funded. Hospitals are exhorted to 'pace themselves' (with too little money) when it comes to non-urgent (which may mean semi-urgent) cases. Thus, towards the end of the financial year, money may be released in lumps for what, in the old NHS, was called the 'tarmacing drives' syndrome.

But overall, too often resources are not allocated 'up front', to allow clinical managers to allocate them at the right time. This may seem a marginal problem but, at the margin, patients are waiting for beds in overbooked surgical wards.

And meanwhile, hospitals work themselves into a worsened version of the old NHS 'efficiency trap', whereby they do much more, more efficiently, at greater value but higher total cost (nowadays, at the same or lower cost, itself too high, given the cuts being imposed specifically upon the hospital sector). So purchasers hammer them. And if they seek to avoid the 'trap', then they are hammered for turning away patients.

A separate purchaser may well be an agency which seeks to maximise its power and influence (the 'bureau shaping' model) – why do we assume providers should be healthily nasty and selfish but not purchasers? The reformers were naive about how to use public choice theory. More specifically, creating the purchaser creates an agency which in practice is interfering with the smooth flow of funds for patient care. Furthermore, GP fundholders, for example, are sometimes duplicating hospital services (with day-care units). Admittedly some A&E initiatives from fundholders send the incentives the right way – less workload for hospitals and more triage. But overall the purchaser/provider split is wasting resources which could fund more, or higher quality, patient care.

Under the rhetoric of a 'primary care-led NHS' and 'health promotion', the government loads onto the NHS the responsibility which the whole range of social policy ought to carry. Of course, we believe in preventing ill health rather than the NHS simply being an illness service. But there is still a requirement for an illness service and the illness service cannot have its budget swallowed up by using the NHS budget to deal with growing social inequality, unemployment, homelessness, environmental problems, antismoking campaigns and dangerous roads. Yet valuable resources are eaten up in creating large bureaucracies (broadly around commissioning and purchasing) which debate 'healthy alliances' while new hospital wards are mothballed due to lack of resources. In one English city, the main teaching hospital has been described by its chief executive as merely an emergency service (if that), while the health authority employs 27 health promotion officers. One should not be blaming the health promotion officers, of course: it is a question of the government passing the buck to the NHS for the health of the nation as well as for ensuring adequate hospital care for the nation.

Would it not make more sense to devise (or re-devise) a system which recognises existing demand at the door, most of which is based upon need in any case? Hospitals and other services could then be funded in anticipation of workload and the more sensible location for this funding would be at the regional level. All the bureaucratic spawn surrounding commissioning could then be replaced with a robust system in which need, and flows of patients, were modelled and predicted, with hospitals and other services being funded accordingly. If you must use the language of a purchaser/provider split, the region would be the purchaser and hospitals and other services would be the provider. There would be scope for a 'bare bones' district health team to ensure appropriate co-ordination of hospital and non-hospital services.

But trends up to 1997 have arguably got it completely wrong. The region became merely a regional office, whereas the challenge ought to be to create greater representation and legitimacy at the regional level, which is where the most crucial planning decisions ought to be taken. This does not mean a large regional health authority, but a robust and strategic one. Labour may seek such an approach in a second term, but the signs are that regional planning will remain tacit at first.

With the growth of rhetoric about locality purchasing in the context of a primary care-led NHS, we are witnessing the birth of bureaucracy at purchaser level just as governments were seeking to eradicate some of this at provider level (first through Mr Heseltine's 'bumf-busters' at the NHS efficiency unit, later through Labour's mergers policy).

Getting rid of 'extracontractual referrals', which have been identified as one of the greatest sources of waste of management time, out of proportion to the cases involved, is of course difficult as ECRs are part of the logic of the new system. However, automatically funding them is the only way to get rid of them without bureaucracy. Otherwise agreeing protocols as to what is and is not an ECR will simply create purchaser/GP labyrinths and bureaucracies.

Tinkering with the current system is rather like punching the balloon – if you want to get rid of a swelling at one part, you are likely to create an equal swelling elsewhere. Unfortunately all of this has little to do with increased allocative or technical efficiency; and a lot to do with the unplanned bureaucratic 'fall-out' of ill thought out policy. The ultimate consequences will be less money for patient care; more pressure on the service; lower morale within the service; and the erosion of a once fine NHS through a mixture of conspiracy and cock-up.

If we really want individuals to choose their health care, as consumers, it would be simpler to give them vouchers rather than create Kafka-esque systems of surrogate purchasing. But even when funded from public money, of course, a voucher system would erode the NHS as we know it, despite egalitarian commentators arguing for similar approaches. (The so-called 'prudent insurance principle' says, 'Ask individuals what they'd insure for – and not insure for – given their own money'. But choices would depend on social class and setting. Again, people would use their vouchers to deal with their overall social problems.)

But in any case governments are not really concerned about genuine public participation: they are more interested in legitimising inevitable decisions which flow from current health policy and levels of funding. It is another form of buck passing. The public in effect have to lump it, so let's persuade them that they are lumping it through their own choice.

The reality of health planning is that economies of scale as well as assurance of adequate clinical quality, in the context of a strictly cash-limited service, constrain 'local choice' to a huge extent.

As a result, encouraging 'Local Voices' can become a bit of a joke. We all know from Sir Humphrey Appleby that opinion polls can be used to prove anything. Popular choice is often intransitive – meaning that a majority may prefer A to B, a majority may prefer B to C, yet a majority prefers C to A. Apply that to medical care and you simply cannot have a list of preferences in order of priority to be 'purchased'. (The reason for the intransitivity is, of course, that the majority is composed of different people from within the total population on each occasion.)

Rationing procedures only provide part of the answer. They involve controversial value judgements, of course. For example, devices such as the QALY do not allow individuals to decide what the benefits of a particular medical procedure are in their own case. They simply take some kind of social average and use that to define a standard 'utility' from each procedure, which can then be set against the cost. Yet this may bear no relation to how individuals, either subjectively or in light of their wider social relationships with family and others, value such procedures. In the language of welfare economics, the QALY is based on interpersonal comparisons of utility. Now since we cannot poll the whole nation on establishing an order of priorities for health care (and if we did, incidentally, it would make a bit of a mockery of local voices), we are using contested means of deciding upon utilities. Even if we make QALYs more sophisticated by differentiating benefit from different medical procedures according to age, social class and so forth, we still cannot overcome the fact that some of us are judging the prospects of others. This may be considered inevitable.

The Oregon approach to rationing has run into severe problems as a result of this and produces some allegedly unacceptable and untenable conclusions as a result – dental capping coming out higher than treating appendicitis, for example. Such schemes will never be robust when it comes to matters of 'life and death': in this sense, health care is exceptional and if we ration out certain procedures contentiously, we will allow those who can afford it to buy it privately.

In any case, medical care is not a technical 'given'. Procedures have different risks and benefits. Individuals rate risks and benefits differently. Thus before one even considers the denominator of cost, it may be that one individual would choose a procedure where the favourable outcome is higher in benefit than with the alternative procedure but where it carries greater risk, and vice versa.

QALYs are ironically opposed by those clinicians who stress the individual patient and also by certain egalitarians who object to the utilitarian bias of a system which simply tots up widgets of health outcome rather than looking at broader distributive issues and issues of equalisation as well as maximisation. The best defenders of the QALY argue, quite rightly, that if there has to be real rationing, one can use the QALY simply as a means of allowing the public to make choices. At its best, this is the QALY's purpose.

We ought to recognise that public wants are shaped by the sense of the possible and available and that to some extent 'the public wants what the public gets'. Purchasers/commissioners of health care are by and large conduits for government policy, concerning process rather than outcomes, charters rather than health achievements.

Is it not time to create one system for the NHS instead of the many? Currently we have a part-market; a part-bureaucracy; a panoply of purchasers and providers within inadequately defined roles; and a growing tension between local choice and national diktat. All of this is spawning a huge bureaucracy where one leg does not know what the other is doing.

Cut to large city hospital. Recently constructed ward mothballed due to financial problems. When enough fundholders can club together to generate two days' work, the ward is opened for minor surgery patients and overspill patients from elsewhere who can fit in temporarily on the days the ward happens to be open. It is rather like a charter flight – it can take off when enough seats have been filled. Equipment is stored in unused sections of the ward and some beds are still mothballed. Lunch and dinner are bought-in cellophane sandwiches (with an apple after dinner).

The patient who has waited six months before getting an initial outpatient appointment and then has heard nothing for nine months after the initial outpatient consultation is asked to come in at one and a half days' notice. Many of the patients on that ward are in this situation. They are patients of fundholders who find money available towards the end of the financial year, so they come in and get done as part of the job lot.

Meanwhile, hospitals are forced to break even annually and make a 6% rate of return on capital. Capital charges rise but income does not. Hospitals which invest face perverse incentives; hospitals which preserve high labour force costs as an alternative may also be squeezed.

This is the kind of NHS which was created by a combination of fundholding and short-termist marketing by trusts, especially those in financial difficulties. It was an understandable dynamic of the system. 'Regulating away' such arbitrariness is the approach of the Labour government after 1997. But such dynamics have a dynamic of their own.

7 The future

AN ALTERNATIVE POLICY

If one links concluding observations to recommendations for the future, then it would be important to 'economise on transactions costs but retain incentives for more efficient performance' (Robinson and Le Grand, in Saltman and von Otter, 1995). Given that NHS providers have a high proportion of fixed costs and stable links with local populations, it becomes important to define criteria of performance. It is also important to restrict opportunistic behaviour by providers who behave as if they are operating in a fiercely competitive market but are in fact reacting to an amalgam of perverse incentives – those deriving from financial squeeze from above and those deriving from the need to shift costs to other providers.

It would be impractical and expensive to get around the alleged problem of limited competition by the paradox of regulation to increase competition, exemplified by the view that 'if there is a local monopoly, then break it up'. In practice, this may well mean breaking up integrated services and co-operative relationships between providers which are eminently sensible. Such a 'pro-competitive' policy has its origin in the search for alternatives to monopoly and utilities but, whatever its applicability there, it is not sensibly applicable to the National Health Service. The approach of Labour after 1997 – mergers and rationalisation – sounded the death knell for such ideological genuflections.

Instead, having experienced the costs of fragmentation, it is important to seek to retain some of the 'micro' benefits of the reforms where they exist (often due to the 'Hawthorne' effect and local management initiative in a climate of uncertainty) yet within a more integrated system with clearer policy priorities as well as clearer service priorities.

Whether one calls the desired model for the NHS 'public competition' or a planned service, there may be some savings available from actually increasing patient choice (expressed through free GP referral, as existed in the old system) and more global service agreements which are less expensive to arrange and police. That is, contracting (implying two sides to a contract) could be replaced with more aggregate, long-term funding linked to GPs' desired referrals and quantified predicted workload. This can be modified over time. Such a system is planning, not competition.

Currently, interpreted at least partly at the political level, there has been investment both in senior management and in the control of senior management through short-term contracts and performance-related pay (related to government objectives) in the hope that more can be squeezed out of the system. In practice, this has often meant intensification of labour and lower wages for the economically and politically weaker cadres within the health service. One man's efficiency gain in this context is another man's exploitation. There are aspects of 'reprofiling the workforce' and 're-engineering the total business' in providers which involve creativity and innovation, undoubtedly. More appropriate use of skills and more appropriate co-ordination of the mix of skills around the patient are important. It is equally important, however, to do so in the context of positive incentive. Currently, as elsewhere in the public sector, keeping one's job or avoiding a pay cut is the best on offer.

Concerning the co-ordination of the service, co-ordinating providers' activities without excessive bureaucracy is important. Unless one is obsessed with the Holy Grail of the purchaser/provider split, the health authority is the body to do this. 'Market' trusts need to be reintegrated into the realm of public purpose. At the same time, providers should retain their identity, for example to prevent a blurring of hospital and community functions and units. But it is costly to regulate for co-operation, having ironically already reduced it by excessive disaggregation and encouragement of market behaviour. Better to move to long-term service agreements funded from a high enough tier to avoid excessive bureaucracy in 'purchasing' – say, democratised regions. This would leave the health authority as the (hopefully lean) co-ordinator of local providers. Many providers are being, and should be, merged, to allow savings to add to those obtained from long-term service agreements rather than short-term contracts.

There is no need for separate non-executive boards for every trust (in addition to the boards of health authorities). They often get in the way of rationalisation, in any case. Thus, an authority with local representatives would be a co-ordinator of local providers, yet providers could retain the direct link between workload and finance which the reforms were supposed to allow, by being funded from region. And greater legitimacy for the public health service would be established or restored. Currently the public feels alienated from a highly centralised NHS. Only general elections allow input by the public. Every other tier is either civil servants (regional offices), quangos (health authorities and trusts) or unelected GP fundholders.

To sum up, a more economical and yet also efficient system would be: regional funding; provider self-management; yet accountability of providers to health authorities, to ensure co-ordination of care. 'Local needs' would be represented at region, to combine representation and effective planning.

Finally, it is important to remember that structural change involved in 'reforming the reforms' is likely to have worthwhile but limited impact. As always, it is true that 'the Chancellor can save more lives than the NHS', as a recent press release for the Association of Public Health put it. Poverty and other social and environmental factors are major influences on health.

That said, it is important to find both institutional and behavioural means of eradicating some of the perverse incentives identified in this and other studies. It is important to minimise the costs associated with short-termism in contracting; over-institutionalisation of the purchaser/provider split; and attempts to operationalise a market when its benefits are unlikely to be realised for a variety of reasons. 'Overdevolution' of purchasing has incurred huge transactions costs yet the real planning 'teeth' are at a higher level in any case.

If the reforms have produced both unintended consequences (such as high administrative and transactions costs) and intended but unwelcome consequences (such as adversarial relationships), does it make any sense to go back to the drawing board? For both managers and professionals, 'reform fatigue' has set in. Ironically, the more the reforms have been debilitating, the less can yet more change be contemplated without nightmares, whatever the consequences of the reforms. One can add to this the political perception by the then Labour opposition, rightly or wrongly, that there must be 'no turning back' – a sort of pale pink version of Mrs Thatcher's Tina (There Is No Alternative). As a result, talk has been of 'reforming the reforms' rather than reversing them. The 1992 election was the last time the latter seemed on the cards and we have subsequently learned from Neil Kinnock that even that was an illusion (Timmins, 1996). By 1997, Labour was conservative, rather than 'old' radical.

Nevertheless, there is reform and reform. Just as both the 'Griffiths changes' and the reforms were overtly claimed by government not to be reorganisations, there is scope for change which benefits the majority of health service actors without involving bureaucratic reorganisation mandated by manuals the size of telephone directories. (The 1974 reorganisation and associated new planning mechanisms spawned the 'Blue and Grey Books' which still live in the institutional memory of the service!)

On this argument, improvements should:

- be geared to reintegrating the NHS, to minimise perverse incentives and adversarial relationships, as well as to reduce the costs of administering (the word is chosen deliberately) the short-termist market;
- constitute a planning tier with visibility and legitimacy at regional level, with responsibility *inter alia* for specialist services and for rationalising services which are served by populations beyond the boundaries of health authorities. This authority may derive legitimacy from regional government or (in the absence of such) from appointments reflecting the skills and interests of the community;
- ensure that providers are funded from region as the result of a planning process which involves considerations of access and equity; trade-off between distance to care, safety and quality; and as much flexibility as possible, to allow for continuing innovation and technological development. Despite the rhetoric of free marketeers, this approach, if handled properly, can be much less 'bureaucratic' than the managed market. Such a planning process will involve key actors such as clinicians, GPs and nurses as well as 'planning experts' such as epidemiologists, social geographers, etc.

A key question is, at what level should planning be undertaken, in the sense of siting and resiting services? The regional tier should do some; the health authority tier should be responsible for intra-authority services. Representatives of groups such as GPs should be involved at either tier, according to interests and abilities, but sparingly. Otherwise the management costs of the market system will be replicated bureaucratically. For example, GP representatives at regional level can advise on acceptability of travel times, availability of A&E and so forth. At health authority level, they can advise on quality of discharge processes, hospital and community service co-operation and so forth.

One result of the reforms has been the loss of appropriate planning for appropriate sizes of population. National and regional services require supra-health authority planning. District services require supra-local, or supra-GP, planning. Of course, as technology changes, 'appropriate' national, regional, district and local services change. And it is not just a technical process – within available resources, choices have to be made between (for example) proximity to care for patients and economies of scale, allowing a greater quantum of service overall (or even higher quality, high specification and expertise). But planning for different levels of service should be done for populations not too large to prevent services being targeted on those who need them and not too small to prevent wild (statistical) variations annually in need and use. For different types of service, different tiers are needed.

Once such planning is done, natural communities require co-ordination of services – another loss associated with the reforms. Health authorities (by any other name) are needed to manage links between hospitals, community services and GPs.

What about the purchaser/provider split? A major function of the health authority should be to co-ordinate local providers. This does not prevent the same authority from planning locally. Whether or not providers have boards is a matter arguably for local choice, which should also dictate what such boards are for. In the absence of market contracting, boards may have less of a role. On the other hand, they may be a useful source of audit for the management of the provider. If one wishes to retain the language of the purchaser/provider split, it is merely (but importantly) a distinction between planning and managing. Separating these organisationally in order to run a market can, however, prevent plans from being carried out appropriately.

- unify capital planning, including decisions about investing and disinvesting in services, with recurrent funding (running costs). Since the reforms, the former has been centralised, not least owing to the Private Finance Initiative and the politics of operating it, while the latter has been decentralised. GP fundholder groups, for example, have no influence on planning, but the power to withhold revenue from planned services. This is, again, an exacerbation of a problem in the old NHS which occurred when the revenue consequences of capital decisions taken at region were not honoured or agreed at district. Now the problem is that local purchasing (contracting) may contradict either actual or desired planning (rationalisation of services, in the main, in a fiscally cold climate) undertaken at a higher level (in the regional office of the NHS executive or even by ministers themselves in reality).

It would be more sensible to involve those, such as fundholders, who currently spend money at too low a level to allow rational and co-ordinated service planning and funding, in the planning process *per se* or, in the interests of manageability, their representatives. They would then be free to refer patients to services without the bureaucracy of contracting, etc. Thus a major advantage of the pre-reform NHS would be combined with more sensitive service planning, some of which flows from greater GP involvement after the reforms (admittedly by necessity in many cases, to protect their patients' interests in the era of contracting and the end to 'free referral').

Services would be funded not by contract but by global cost. This of course necessitates accurate costing (although not at the level of per patient) but, as the history of NHS costing shows long before the reforms, this is not the same as a marketplace with its contracting. When some have recently advocated longer term contracting (three or five years, instead of annual), the objection has been raised that the annual public expenditure round prohibits it. This ironically is an objection to precise, quasi-legal contracting; it was never a problem in the old NHS, where changes in public expenditure prognosis simply had to be absorbed. (Or rather, it was a problem, in that greater long-term clarity was desirable then as now, but it was not a formal 'constitutional' problem.)

Instead, predicted need would lead to allocations to hospitals and other providers. If referral patterns, technology and/or costs changed over time, so be it. Planning is iterative. Global allocations to adequately large institutions, over adequate time periods, make adjustment easier. Indeed, a major problem with the reforms has been short-term, over-rigid contracts with many fragmented trusts. Virement has been difficult (although 'poaching' of cash has also been more difficult, arguably imposing more discipline).

If there is not enough cash in the system to finance referrals, admissions and emergencies as prevailing, it is also part of the planning exercise to take the tough decisions. In that sense, the difference between the old NHS, the post-reform NHS and any new alternative is simply how this is done. Is it best done informally, managerially or 'democratically'? One thing is clear: again, both health authorities and regions need to be involved. The problem with *Local Voices* is that it has raised a false prospectus: firstly, local choices may not be tenable financially, as part of the bigger picture (i.e. decision making is devolved too low, on many issues); and, secondly, fundholding GPs may not make decisions which tally with health authority, let alone regional, perceived agendas or needs.

THE FUTURE FINANCING OF THE NHS

The NHS reforms began as a political reaction to perceived underfunding in the NHS. It is therefore worth reviewing the prospects for the future types and level of financing of the National Health Service.

Firstly, publicly financed and publicly provided health services have a good record in combining a reasonable level of equity, economy and effectiveness in targeting services at the 'macro' level. Efficiency, and not merely economy, at the 'micro' level is also high (by international standards) in the National Health Service, although there is debate, not least around the reforms themselves, as to whether market mechanisms improve or decrease such efficiency.

Secondly, if Britain is to compete in the increasingly internationalised capitalist world economy (it is often assumed or argued), an economy characterised by low taxation and low public expenditure is necessary. This implies severe pressure on finance for the NHS. There are of course alternative approaches: a 'high investment' approach is possible and challenges to the current system of international capital flows and international trade are possible using supranational blocs. This is not the place to debate such issues.

Nevertheless the most appropriate means of raising finance is an important issue. It is often claimed that if public health care, or extra public health care, is unaffordable, then those who are able to do so ought to provide for themselves privately. This argument is often based on a fallacy. If indeed public 'single payer' financing of health care is more efficient and less administratively costly, then not only is it advantageous for the 'better off' to be insured or provided for publicly, but there may also as a result be a slight dividend to allow such a public insurance or taxation policy to be redistributive. This same argument applies in so-called poor countries, including developing countries and the countries of former Eastern Europe. If there is 'no money' for public health services, how can it be assumed that there is money to be mobilised for private payment or private self-insurance by the better off? This argument only obtains if public health services are seen as politically undesirable or impossible (such that, for example, people wish to insure themselves privately, even if less efficiently) or if it is assumed that public insurance is less efficient. The international evidence points in a contrary direction.

It is often pointed out that extra money can only be mobilised through private sources or private insurance. This also may be a misconception. If the system of taxation and public expenditure prevailing has become more regressive, then even if the same percentage of GDP is spent on health and indeed on other public services, the amount of money left in private hands 'after tax' may be proportionately more in the hands of the better off. As a result, there will be more consumption of private health care or private health insurance, in all likelihood. A more progressive system of taxation (which is also more likely to be associated with policies which diminish health inequalities more generally) is capable of mobilising extra money for the health sector. This is not, of course, to underestimate the political difficulties involved in so doing. That is why ideas have been revived recently for an 'earmarked' (or hypothecated) tax, the proceeds from which would go specifically to health.

Equally, comparing Britain with other countries in terms of the public/private mix in health-care financing may also be misleading. It is pointed out (for example) that The Netherlands, although spending a considerably higher percentage of GDP on health care, does so through mobilising more private money. Much of this, however, is statutory contribution to public insurance, which is in effect public taxation by any other name.

Many schemes of 'public insurance' around the world indeed obey the principles of taxation rather than the principles of insurance and are simply an earmarked form of taxation, with the proceeds going specifically to health (whether administered as part of the social security scheme or health specific). That is, when one gets away from words and names and when one considers the similarities between public insurance and public taxation, it can be seen that Britain spends relatively little by comparison with comparable countries even on public care, not just on the total of health-care financing.

Once the level of financing has been decided, the challenge is to ensure that financing is mobilised as efficiently and effectively as possible, although of course the two issues are related, in that the type of system chosen may have implications for the level of spending, as a result of longer term political consequences of the system chosen. Again, there is international evidence that the public, 'single payer' model is capable of being administratively efficient and of directing resources to national priorities more effectively and directly than alternative systems. Such assertions are of course incapable of definitive proof and rely on a variety of indirect evidence.

Next, ensuring efficiency in provision and in the links between financing and provision (including purchasing and provision, in the language of the new NHS) is important. Here we reach a central debate around the NHS reforms.

Consider the following simple typology of health-care systems.

1. Broadly private systems, relying on private finance and private fee-for-service provision (of which the US is the dominant example).
2. European systems relying on broadly public insurance yet decentralised and largely fee-for-service provision.
3. More integrated European systems, broadly relying on public taxation and more integrated public provision (as in Britain, even after the reforms, and Sweden) (Paton, 1996).

It is worth asking, what constitutes health sector reform? For countries in categories one and two above, a movement to a public 'internal market' model may in fact represent improvements in efficiency as well as in equity. For a largely private system, moving to more integrated financing and larger scale contracting with providers may increase both equity and efficiency. For the 'expensive' European systems in category two, the systems of contracting represented by the NHS's internal market may in fact lead to a reduction in administrative costs, or at least no increase, as well as an increase in allocative efficiency due to more overt purchasing according to need. This is especially true if the same level of financing is preserved.

It is, however, a misconception to imply that countries in category three will benefit from converting their relatively integrated public systems to the market model, for they may significantly increase their administrative costs without commensurate benefit in allocative efficiency. The challenge for such countries is therefore to improve incentives for efficiency and effectiveness at the 'micro' level without creating the institutions and perverse incentives associated with imperfectly functioning markets.

That is, for countries such as Britain, health sector reform should consist in preserving equity (and indeed, extending it where possible) and increasing efficiency in an appropriate manner, without adopting the 'solutions' which countries in categories one and two may increasingly seek to adopt.

If one conceptualises a continuum of health-care systems from the largely private to the integrated public, appropriate heath sector reform within already integrated public systems may involve more efficient and effective planning mechanisms and structures with more appropriate reimbursement of providers in terms of relating resources to workload. On this interpretation, the British reforms may have been a sledgehammer to crack a nut. Maintaining the integrated nature of the NHS while improving allocative efficiency and appropriate funding of providers was the challenge for the NHS. At the time of the reforms, the ideological thrust behind them may have prevented appropriate consideration of the full range of options.

Health sector reform in comparable European countries is taking diverse routes. In Sweden, earlier interest in copying the British model waned after the election of a Social Democratic government in late 1994. In The Netherlands, health sector reform (based on increased competition between purchasers as well as providers and also an attempt to define a national 'core' level of services below the level of those currently reimbursed publicly) was significantly stymied in the 1990s. In the US, from a very different direction, the Clinton reforms – broadly to increase equity, co-ordinate purchasing and use market mechanisms in provision, although potentially with very high administrative costs – were also stymied. Once again, US politics prevented a constituency for reform being translated into action (Mann and Ornstein, 1995; Paton, 1990).

The last thing the health service in Britain seemed to want in 1997 was another major administrative upheaval inadequately addressed to real problems. However, this should not prevent the alteration in a practical manner of inappropriate or destructive aspects of the 'reformed NHS'. The overall watchword presumably ought to be a combination of equity, efficiency and effectiveness. This requires a streamlining of financing, of provision and of the links between the two. That is the direction in which the reforms ought to be 'reformed'. In other words, excessive cost without commensurate benefit in purchasing ought to be diminished (as explored below). Excessive disaggregation and fragmentation, in provision, with the perverse incentives engendered as a result, ought to be tackled. Current malfunctioning of the purchaser/provider split, as well as currently excessive costs in rendering that split operational, ought also to be tackled.

A PESSIMISTIC SCENARIO FOR DEFENDERS OF A COMPREHENSIVE NHS

Just as the reforms were a complex package of policies with often unintended consequences, they were also part of a wider set of policies which are still changing the NHS, gradually but significantly. If current trends in fiscal, social and health policy continue, then the NHS will face increasing pressure over the coming years and a comprehensive, universal service of adequate quality will be a bridge too far. The reforms were not the source of this, but they provided mechanisms which facilitated it. The following paragraphs seek to explain.

Economic change in Britain since the 1980s has produced two effects highly relevant to the future of the welfare state. Firstly, after-tax income is proportionately more in the hands of the better off. (That is, the tax system has become less progressive, alongside economy-wide changes in income differentials before tax.) Secondly, profit levels have risen significantly: for example, dividends have risen from 1.5% to 5.4% of GDP since 1980.

As a result, to spend the same money in real terms, or the same percentage of GDP, on the welfare state means to tax the less well off proportionately more. Added to this, there is a tendency on the part of the better off to spend a bit more privately, from higher disposable incomes, on goods such as education and health. Extra private spending (or insurance) on health in Britain has been noted since 1980, although to a more modest extent than on many other goods given the existence of an NHS to which virtually the whole nation subscribes both culturally and politically.

The more the better off spend privately, it is sometimes argued, the more there is left for the poorer within public budgets such as the NHS's. This, however, is a static view. Private consumption of welfare goods tends to be transacted more expensively. There is therefore further political resistance to tax, or increased tax revolt, on the part of the better off. Instead of paying publicly for, say, a comprehensive, universal NHS, which allows richer taxpayers to pay for themselves and also redistribute a modest amount to others, they now find themselves spending the same without any element of redistribution. (That is, they pay less tax, for a more basic NHS, plus more privately.) To generate the same budget for the NHS, let alone growth over time, therefore means more tax burden on the poorer, which include, for these purposes, lower to middle-income earners. The poorer also therefore are susceptible to the lure or siren of tax revolt, as they find themselves proportionately more burdened by tax.

As a result, there is more pressure on the NHS budget. Add to this the second element above, the need for higher profit – partly political choice, partly the corollary of living in the world economy where attracting inward investment is the name of the game, in an age when the power of capital *vis-à-vis* both national governments and labour has hugely increased. The need to offer high profit calls not only for low taxes and low public expenditure, but the use of that public expenditure, in part, to support the profitability of the economy. This in turn not only gives more impetus to shifting the cost of health care, etc. from employers and the better off to workers and citizens generally, but also calls for a lower wage bill in the health service as the search for increased economy-wide profit turns to workers generally and to health workers in particular. The latter are a factor of production in an 'industry' which in part has the function of investing in a healthy workforce.

The twin effects are therefore more regressive financing of health care and greater exploitation of health workers (a term which includes professionals, of course). So far, nothing has been said of the institutions and incentives created by the NHS reforms. They may, however, be used to facilitate such a process, not necessarily as the result of some grand conspiracy but through a process of adaptation and realisation of their potential as they evolve.

Firstly, the reforms created a market mechanism (if not a market), the principal use (and indeed justification) of which is to force down providers' costs through a competitive contracting process. The largest component of providers' costs is labour. Efficiency savings therefore target work practices, but also seek to squeeze the maximum out of the minimum labour (whether doctors or cleaners).

Secondly, the contracting process encourages purchasers to seek deals at marginal or low cost. In their eagerness to cement deals, financially strapped providers often make contracts at rates which are unsustainable in the long term. Often such deals are centrally prompted or ordered, as with 'waiting list initiatives' which would only be sustainable if 'one-off' money, provided for one year, were recurrent (in an age when there is little fat left to squeeze from the system, yet a ministerial pretence that efficiency savings do not affect patient care). In our case studies of providers in the West Midlands Region, the unsustainability of the waiting list initiatives of 1994–95 was a frequent refrain.

As a result, capital as well as labour is squeezed, in the NHS, through the contracting process. (It could be done by direct command, but a combination of market incentive and political fiat is effective.)

The more 'ordinary citizens' finance their own NHS care in a less progressive tax system, the more they will seek to pass on the hardship to NHS employees, i.e. to get as much as possible from a more directly impacting budget. Of course, as with all industries, citizens can be users/consumers and workers together. When prices are cut or, in the case of a public service, the costs of providing it are cut, do people gain more as consumers than they lose as workers? Again, a dynamic picture must be sought: different groups of employees will gain or lose differentially, depending upon how their industry's wages, profits and prices change and how such changes are augmented or counteracted by changes in other industries. For example, if the wage bill is halved in a factory, is all the 'benefit' passed on to consumers or is it wholly or partially passed on to higher profits? And, for those workers whose wages are halved, are the prices (or costs through tax of public services) they confront elsewhere commensurately halved or not? That is, does the process occur in a standard manner or is it differential?

In practice, there may be a 'hierarchy of exploitation' whereby there is, in most industries, a shift from wages to profits (the degree varies, industry to industry). Some workers (the weakest) lose more than they gain in lower prices/costs elsewhere (lower prices are possible, as savings on wages may be shared between a firm's consumers and profit-takers) and some workers (the strongest) gain more from others' wage cuts than they lose from their own.

The effect of this political economy in recent years has been to place increasing stress on the NHS (as well as other welfare services). Hard-pressed taxpayers are in effect participating in a politically mandated zero-sum game with NHS workers, summed up by ministers as consumers versus vested interests (i.e. workers).

Hospital trusts, increasingly facing financial deficits, annually and alone (without the chance of budgetary virement, after the reforms' strict contractual categories), and increasingly facing 'bankrupt' purchasers, could only seek to obey charters concerning elective admissions (from many separate purchasers) and to admit emergencies as well by further stripping and squeezing the workforce. This may then endanger appropriate patient care and appropriate discharge. The media, by 1996–97, was increasingly finding both hospital chief executives and regional office directors to comment on how close their various systems were coming to breaking point.

None of this required the reforms to happen, but they have their role in the picture. And seeking savings in 'management costs', fine in theory, may be difficult if the relevant managers were hired to police the labyrinth of the 'reformed' NHS and (at the top level) at high salaries and on short-term contracts, consonant with giving the incumbents a vested interest in defence of the new system and obedience to its progenitors. Management cuts, in this context, are more likely to mean more squeeze upon middle managers at the sharp end.

In the 1990s, neither main political party developed policy consonant with the problems facing the NHS. Indeed, the new orthodoxy was likely to deepen problems. Many of the administrative costs of the purchaser/provider split, with or without GP fundholding, were likely to remain. The Private Finance Initiative became more acceptable to the Labour Party (albeit in technically different form), as Labour accepted Conservative spending plans up to 2002, preventing public investment on any significant scale.

As a result, private investment for new hospitals, for example, could lead to (not so much creeping but overt) privatisation. The purchaser/provider split had led to 'autonomous' trusts and private capital as the main source of their development meant they were *de facto* private providers. Private investors require profit and thus funds from the future revenue budget of the NHS are needed to 'pay back' private capital, plus profit. Private capital is not a free good and the drying up of public capital (simply but unproclaimed) means the future use of revenue budgets for capital costs. (Public capital was to be cut 22% between 1994 and 1999.)

When one adds limits on public expenditure affecting the total NHS budget, increased private spending (outside the NHS) can be predicted (with all its long-term effects, described above) alongside increased private provision. An alternative, optimistic scenario (for defenders of a public NHS) would require political and fiscal will currently in short supply. Judgement on the new government after 1997 will include such matters.

THE LABOUR GOVERNMENT'S WHITE PAPER, *THE NEW NHS: MODERN AND DEPENDABLE*

On Tuesday 9th December 1997, the Labour Government published its White Paper for the National Health Service, entitled *The New NHS: Modern and Dependable*. In the foreword, the Prime Minister, Tony Blair, stated that 'creating the NHS was the greatest act of modernisation ever achieved by a Labour Government'. Given the importance laid upon the term 'modernisation' by New Labour, this was an important statement. For defining the NHS *per se* as modernisation meant that it was less likely to be subjected to the sort of fundamental review instigated for other aspects of the welfare state and consisting primarily in 'hard choices' (principally redistribution within static budgets, 'from the poor to the poor').

At the political level, Labour's agenda was to combine a reintegration of the NHS (after the fragmentation of the internal market) with an allegedly forward-looking policy which meant 'no turning back' to the 1970s and the situation prior to 18 years of Conservative government. Additional and related to this, there was a desire to avoid another fundamental structural reorganisation. Whether or not there was an actual need for the latter, permanent revolution under the Conservatives had ironically helped entrench the Conservative reforms by removing any appetite for further significant change. A further requirement of Labour's new policy was that administrative costs were to be cut in order to allow more resources for 'front line' patient care.

Thus to a certain extent, 'old radicalism' (the socialism that dare not speak its name under New Labour) was to have more of a place in the pantheon of the NHS than elsewhere in society – but was to be linked to an alleged new pragmatism, if not new radicalism, which looked to the future. At one level, of course, this was the politics of the soundbite. If everything has to be 'new', then simply defining the emergent policy as 'new' is the means to achieve it!

At the level of political overview, the internal market was to be abolished and GP fundholding was to be superseded. Yet the purchaser/provider split (now justified in Labour's language as merely the distinction between commissioning and service management) was to remain. The main change was that commissioning – seemingly synonymous with purchasing – was now to be entrusted to Primary Care Groups (PCGs), rather than Health Authorities. Health Authorities themselves were expected to become fewer in number through mergers over time and were to take ultimate responsibility for planning services (that is, for strategic decisions as to closing hospitals, merging hospitals and building new services). Yet Primary Care Groups, typically representing populations of around 100,000 and comprising around 50 GPs, community nurses and possibly other actors, were to be the actual purchasers.

One of the purposes of these groups was to seek to achieve a single unified budget for funding for all hospital and community services, prescribing and general practice infrastructure. It was no doubt hoped that this would lead to more effective and efficient use of resources, primarily by giving GPs responsibility for the 'seamless' and integrated care of patients.

Another source of the policy to create Primary Care Groups was of course the political motivation to avoid conflict with GPs. It was believed that existing fundholders – especially large groups of fundholders, or consortia holding the total budget for hospital and community services – would see the new policy as an extension of their desired freedom without some of the disadvantages. Making all GPs responsible for commissioning would also end the criticism that the distinction between fundholding and non-fundholding GPs created a two tier service.

This was nevertheless quite a risky strategy. For non-fundholding GPs, especially those represented by the Association of Commissioning GPs, did not generally want the responsibility of holding budgets. On the other side of the fence, considering fundholders, different reactions were possible. Some fundholders welcomed the Labour Government's White Paper. Others however saw the new policy as taking away their power yet increasing their responsibilities. (And of course there were those fundholders who were not very keen on fundholding, but who had merely become so in order to maximise advantage under the previous government's reforms.)

The ultimate effects of the new White Paper, when passed into legislation, would crucially depend on how much of the power of the Health Authority was being taken by the new Primary Care Groups. In the first instance, there was to be a range of different models of Primary Care Groups. This was, in all likelihood, making a virtue out of necessity (or as the White Paper put it somewhat more optimistically, 'going with the grain'). The Labour Government has inherited a spectrum of commissioning arrangements – ranging from locality commissioning groups (groups of GPs working closely with their health authority to commission services); GP fundholding; multi-funds and total purchasers as an extension of GP fundholding; and other commissioning arrangements. Prior to the White Paper's emergence in December 1997, the Labour Government had announced 42 GP Commissioning Group pilot projects, which were to 'go live' on 1st April 1998. These were to be monitored and evaluated by independent researchers, and were to embrace a number of different approaches to GP commissioning (now called Primary Care Group commissioning, in the White Paper).

Concerning the range of models, there were to be four options for Primary Care Groups. These were:

1. The minimalist role – supporting the health authority in commissioning, and acting only in an advisory capacity.
2. Taking devolved responsibility for managing the budget, but as part of the health authority.
3. Becoming free-standing bodies (but accountable to the health authority), contracting for secondary services.
4. Becoming free-standing bodies as in 3 but with the added responsibility for providing community health services for the population (by implication as an alternative to contracting with community trusts for this purpose).

The White Paper was unclear as to whether the ultimate intention was that all Primary Care Groups would become free-standing bodies – or Primary Care Trusts, as the White Paper called them. Indeed the original intention had been that the pilot projects would be assessed to find the most appropriate model or models in light of the objectives of providing effective care and also reducing administration and management costs by comparison with the previous government's internal market. But there was a sentence in the new White Paper which pointed out that Primary Care Groups '... will be expected to progress along (the spectrum) so that in time all Primary Care Groups assume fuller responsibilities.'

Added to this ambiguity was the possibility that the Health Authority would in fact be the iron hand in a velvet glove. The White Paper (paragraph 4.3) stated that amongst the Health Authority's tasks would be 'deciding on the range and location of health care services for the Health Authority's residents, which should flow from and be part of, the Health Improvement Programme'. This Health Improvement Programme was squarely the responsibility of the Health Authority. If, furthermore, the Health Authority was to decide upon the range and location of health care services, then the role of the Primary Care Groups would be simply to purchase services from already-planned and 'commissioned' sources of provision.

Added to this was the Health Authority's revamped and enhanced responsibility for improving public health. Pending publication of a Green Paper to be entitled, *Our Healthier Nation*, it was stated in the White Paper that the Health Authority would work in partnership with local authorities and others to identify the most important local action to make the most impact upon the health of local people. Again it can be asked: if these crucial decisions are to be taken (quite rightly) by the Health Authority, what if Primary Care Groups wished to commission services out of line with these priorities?

This is the perennial question for the NHS: how can national and higher-tier priorities in pursuit of effective health care and a uniform National Health service be reconciled with local freedoms in choosing priorities generally and services specifically? The different agendas embraced by the Labour Government led it to face both ways on this issue. On the one hand, it wanted to stress local freedom. (Indeed an early paragraph in the White Paper said there will be no return to the 'command and control' of the NHS which had existed before the Conservatives' reforms). On the other hand, they wished to reintegrate the service in pursuit of its truly national status. In theory at least, local choice can undermine this objective if different localities make different choices.

The irony is that the NHS which had existed before the Conservative reforms was characterised by *anything but* 'command and control'. Indeed one of the motivations for the Conservative reforms had been to command and control more effectively! New Labour inherited and enhanced this approach: performance management from above was heavily stressed in the new White Paper, and national commissions to police it were announced.

Additionally, the Labour Government had the objective of diminishing the 'transactions costs' which it defined as the hallmark of the internal market. Devolving purchasing responsibility to Primary Care Groups might well increase transactions costs, or at least prevent their diminution. Five Primary Care Groups within each Health Authority could be characterised as five mini-Health Authorities, replicating functions unnecessarily, not least by employing the kind of staff (albeit on a larger scale) which GP fundholders had been employing. And furthermore, it would be another reorganisation of the NHS in all but name (not that this would matter, if – as with the Conservative reforms throughout the 1980s and early 1990s – the aim was merely to avoid reorganisation at the soundbite level).

The more one enters the detail, the more the ambiguity is raised as to whether the internal market was, in fact, being abolished. If Primary Care Groups had the right to decide where to commission services from Trusts (which were to remain in their post-'NHS reforms' state), then it was a question of theology as to whether the market was abolished or not. Or, to put it the other way around, if market forces had already waned under the Conservative Government before 1997, after their short life between 1992 and around 1995, then the Labour Government was not abolishing something which had already been abolished. Around these questions lies the issue of the purchaser/provider split. To some, you can have a purchaser/provider split without a market (presumably the stance of the Labour Government). To others, however, the purchaser/provider split ensures that there will be at least the sort of market we have had since 1991.

As stated earlier in this book, the Labour Government seems to be squaring the circle by *defining* the abolition of the internal market as the move to longer-term contracting (now re-christened service agreements); the abolition of GP fundholding 'as we had known it'; the outlawing of cost-per-case agreements between purchasers and providers, with their high administrative costs; and the alleged abolition of Extra Contractual Referrals through more refined purchasing. Yet these are technical rather than strategic changes, and the last is arguably unachievable.

The new White Paper bore signs of extreme haste, as evidenced by the form of its drafting and the resort to stark lists of bullet points; a strange mix of technical detail and soundbite; and a blurring of the distinction between innovations inherited from the outgoing Government and new developments. As with the Conservative Government's White Paper, Working for Patients, the devil would be in the detail – much of which was yet to be decided and which would no doubt be decided on the hoof.

Labour's White Paper had affinities with New Labour's approach to many policy areas: its first priority was to be strict about the prospect for extra financing (Labour's additional money for the NHS was no different in all likelihood to what the Conservatives would have provided); and, having appeased the economic orthodoxy of the Treasury, the next priority was to seek to offer a carrot to all main interest groups in health care. A major consequence of the Conservative reforms had been the mushrooming of special interests (fundholders and non-fundholders; hospital clinicians in greater conflict with general practitioners; the new management cadre; *et al.*). Yet the danger now was promises based upon a false prospectus. 'Doctors and nurses' were to be brought back to the centre of decision making – but it was often responsibilities rather than powers that they were to be given – not least for rationing. All services, including prescribing budgets, were now to be cash-limited. On the bright side, stress upon collaboration and the pursuit of what was called integrated care was at least likely to provide one of the bases for 'a new start' for the NHS from a government which had less ideological difficulty in accepting the principles of socialised medicine than had its predecessor.

At the end of the day, the practical questions to be resolved included: whether or not real money for all care would be devolved to groups of GPs operating through Primary Care Groups; and the extent to which all GPs should be involved in decision-making as part of such groups. If one subscribes to the view that the GP is the closest health service decision maker to the patient, then there is a quasi-democratic argument for so devolving budgets. Unfortunately, the management costs of such a policy are likely to be high; and furthermore there is no evidence that GPs are either willing or able to carry out such a fundamental role themselves. Ultimately, such a policy is likely to mean devolution to management agencies operating under the aegis of the Health Authority; and the ultimate outcome of the policy might be more management tinkering rather than a truly innovative policy. As with the previous government's reforms, the main question which arises concerns incentives and whether they are benign or perverse. What are the key incentives embodied in the White Paper, *The New NHS,* and are they likely to bring improved relations between primary care and hospital care on an affordable basis? That question aside, the new arrangements are at least likely to provide a more stable basis for NHS decision making than the predecessor arrangements – as long as there is a fruitful reconciliation of the respective roles of Regions, Health Authorities and Primary Care Groups.

Finally, the politics of the new policy consisted in 'tacking on' the aspiration of collaboration (not competition) to inherited structures which had been designed for competition (New Labour, Old Conservative!). While new Ministers were clear at the general level about their goals, they relied for the detail on senior NHS management, based in the Executive in the Department of Health, who had lived and breathed the previous government's reforms. The previous government had created a Management Executive allegedly to take the NHS both out of politics and traditional Civil Service administration; but had in fact politicised the Management Executive. Now, the new government was relying on a central management cadre which was actually behaving more like traditional civil servants than 'neutral' managers – in keeping what they were used to, dressed up in new language.

References

Please note: Most key government documents are noted in Chapters 2 and 3

Adams, C. B. T. (1995) Ox dons syndrome. *British Medical Journal*, **311**, 1559–62.

Ambler, W. (1996) Does Fundholding Lead to a Two-Tier System? Keele University Centre for Health Planning and Management, MBA dissertation (Unpublished).

Appleby, J., Smith, P., Ranade, W., Little, V. and Robinson, R. (1994) Monitoring managed competition, in *Evaluating the NHS Reforms*, (eds R. Robinson and J. Le Grand), King's Fund, London.

Ashburner, L. (1994) The composition of NHS trust boards. *Health Services Management Research*, **7**(3), 154–64.

Ashburner, L. and Cairncross, L. (1993) Health authority members: continuity or change? *Public Administration*, **71**(3), 357–75.

Ashburner, L., Ferlie, E. and Fitzgerald, L. (1994) Quasi markets and the development of competition in the NHS. 24th PAC Conference, York.

Bain, J. (1991) General practice and the new contract: reactions and impact. *British Medical Journal*, **302** (6786), 1183–6.

Best, G. and Ham, C. (1989) Goodbye rubber stamp image. *Health Service Journal*, **20th April**, 19.

Bevan, G., Holland, W., Maynard, A. and Mays, N. (1988) *Reforming UK Health Care To Improve Health: The Case for Research and Experiment*, United Medical and Dental Schools and Centre for Health Economics, UMDS, London.

Blane, D. (1985) An assessment of the Black Report's explanations of health inequalities. *Sociology of Health and Illness*, **7**(3), 423–5.

Blaxter, M. (1990) *Health and Lifestyles*, Routledge, London.

British Medical Association (1988) Evidence to the government internal review of the National Health Service. *British Medical Journal*, **296**, 1411–18.

British Medical Association (1989) *Special Report on the Government's White Paper, Working for Patients*, BMA, London.

Butler, F. and Pirie, M. (1988) *The Health of Nations*, Adam Smith Institute, London.

Carr-Hill, R. (1987) The inequalities in health debate: a critical review of the issues. *Journal of Social Policy*, **14**(4), 509–42.

Cartwright, A. and O'Brien, M. (1976) Social class variations in the nature of

Cartwright, A. and O'Brien, M. (1976) Social class variations in the nature of G.P. consultations, in *Sociology of the NHS*, (ed. M. Stacey), Sociological Review Monograph No. 22, Keele University.

Central Statistical Office (CSO) (1992) *Social Trends*, HMSO, London.

Coote, A. and Hunter, D. (1996) *New Agenda for Health*, Institute for Public Policy Research, London.

Day, P. and Klein, R. (1987) *Accountabilities: Five Public Services*, Tavistock, London.

Department of Health and Social Security (1980) *Inequalities in Health: Report of a Research Working Group*, (The Black Report), DHSS, London.

Department of Health (1989a) *Working for Patients* (White Paper), Cmnd 555, HMSO, London.

Department of Health (1989b) *Working Papers 1–8* (White Paper) HMSO, London.

Dobson, F. (1997) Speech to NHS Confederation, June.

Enthoven, A. (1985) *Reflections on the Management of the NHS*, Nuffield Provincial Hospitals Trust, London.

Enthoven, A. (1988) *The Theory and Practice of Managed Competition*, North Holland, Amsterdam.

Enthoven, A. (1995) Managed care – managed competition. *British Medical Journal*, **310**, 165.

Flemming, D. and Oppenheimer, P. (1996) Are government spending and taxes too high (or too low)? *National Institute Economic Review*, 31 July.

Fox, A. J. and Shewry, M. C. (1988) New longitudinal insights into relationships between unemployment and mortality. *Stress Medicine*, **4**, 11–19.

Galbraith, J. K. (1992) *The Culture of Contentment*, Sinclair Stevenson, London.

Glennerster, H. and Matsaganis, M. (1994) *Implementing GP Fundholding*, Open University Press, Buckingham.

Goldsmith, J. (1994) *The Trap*, Macmillan, London.

Goodman, A. and Webb, S. (1994) *For Richer, For Poorer*, Institute of Fiscal Studies, Swansea.

Green, D. (1986) *Challenge to the NHS*, Institute of Economic Affairs, London.

Green, D. (1988) *Everyone a Private Patient*, Institute of Economic Affairs Health Unit, London.

Griffiths, R. (1983) *Letter to the Secretary of State* (The Griffiths Inquiry Report), DHSS, London.

Harrison, D. (1996) Involving GPs in Strategic Planning? Keele University Centre for Health Planning and Management, MBA dissertation (unpublished).

Hatcher, P. (1997) The British health reforms, in *Health Care and Reform in Industrialized Countries*, (ed. M. Raffel), Pennsylvania State University Press, Pittsburgh.

Haynes, R. (1991) Inequalities in health and health service use: evidence from the GHS. *Social Science and Medicine*, **33**, 361–8.

Illsley, R. (1955) Social class selection and class difference in relation to stillbirths and infant deaths. *British Medical Journal*, **2**, 1520.

Illsley, R. and Le Grand, J. (1987) The measurement of inequality, in *Economics and Health*, (ed. A. Williams), Macmillan, London.

Jenkins, S. (1995) *Accountable to None: The Tory Nationalisation of Britain*, Hamish Hamilton, London.

Kaletsky, A. (1996) *The Times*, 1 August, p 27.

Kaplan, G. A. (1985) Twenty years of health in Alameda County: a human population laboratory analysis. Paper presented to the Society for Prospective Medicine General Meeting, San Francisco, 24 November.

Keeley, D. (1991) Personal care or the polyclinic? *British Medical Journal*, **302**(6791), 1514–16.

Klein, R. (1991) The politics of change. *British Medical Journal*, **302**(6785), 1102–3.

Klein, R. (1997) *Steering but not Rowing. The Transformation of the Department of Health – A Case Study*, Polity Press, London.

Labour Party (1995) *Renewing the NHS*, John Smith House, London.

Lee, K. and Mills, A. (1982) *Policy Making and Planning in the Health Sector*, Croom Helm, London.

Le Grand, J. (1994) Evaluating the NHS reforms, in *Evaluating the NHS Reforms*, (eds R. Robinson and J. Le Grand), King's Fund, London.

MacIntyre, S. (1986) The patterning of health by social position in contemporary Britain: directions for sociological research. *Social Science and Medicine*, **23**(4), 393–415.

Mann, T. and Ornstein, N. (1995) *Intensive Care: How Congress Shapes Health Policy*, Brookings Institution, Washington DC.

Marmor, T. (1997) Global health policy reform: misleading mythology or learning opportunity? in *Health Policy Reform, National Variations and Globalization*, (eds C. Altenstetter and J. Björkman), Macmillan, London, and St Martin's, New York.

McLachlan, G. and Maynard, A. (1982) *The Public/Private Mix for Health*, Nuffield Trust, London.

Meadows, S. H. (1961) Social class migration and chronic bronchitis. *British Journal of Social Medicine*, **15**, 171.

Moon, G. and Gillespie, R. (eds) (1995) *Society and Health: An Introduction to Social Science for Health Professionals*, Routledge, London.

MORI/Nuffield Provincial Hospitals Trust (1985) *A Review of Surveys Conducted about the NHS* (unpublished).

NAHAT (1994) *Developing Contracting*, Research Paper No.15. NAHAT, Birmingham.

Netherlands Ministry of Health, Welfare and Sports (1995) *Substitute Mortality and Morbidity*, NMHWS, The Hague.

Nettleton, S. (1995) *The Sociology of Health and Illness*, Polity Press, Cambridge.

NHS Executive (1994) *Local Freedoms, National Responsibilities: Regulating the Internal Market*, NHSE, Leeds.

Nichol, D., Ham, C., Hewitt, P. *et al.* (1995) *Healthcare 2000*, Health Services Management Unit, University of Manchester.

OPCS (1986) *Occupational Mortality: Decennial Supplement 1979–1980, 1982–1983*, HMSO, London.

Owen, D. (1985) Keynote address, Institute of Health Services Management annual conference, Coventry (June).

Paton, C. (1990) *US Health Politics: Public Policy and Political Theory*, Avebury, Aldershot.

Paton, C. (1992) *Competition and Planning in the NHS*, 1st edn, Chapman & Hall, London.

Paton, C. (1995) Present dangers and future threats: some perverse incentives in the NHS reforms. *British Medical Journal*, **310**(1), 1245–8.

Paton, C. (1996) *Health Policy and Management: The Healthcare Agenda in a British Political Context*, Chapman & Hall, London.

Ranade, W. (1985) Motives and Behaviours in DHAs. *Public Administration*, **63**(2), 183–200.

Rathwell, T., Godino, J. and Gott, M. (eds) (1995) *Tipping the Balance Towards Primary Health Care*, Avebury, Aldershot.

Redwood, J. (1988) *In Sickness and in Health: Managing Change in the NHS*, Centre for Policy Studies, London.

Redwood, J. and Letwin, O.(1988) *Britain's Biggest Enterprise: Ideas for Radical Reforms of the NHS*, Centre for Policy Studies, London.

Robinson, R. and Le Grand, J. (1994) *Evaluating the NHS Reforms*, King's Fund, London.

RUHBC (1989) *Changing the Public Health. Research Units in Health and Behavioural Change*, John Wiley, Chichester.

Saltman, R. and von Otter, C. (1992) *Planned Markets and Public Competition*, Open University Press, Buckingham.

Saltman, R. and von Otter, C. (eds) (1995) *Implementing Planned Markets in Health Care*, Open University Press, Buckingham.

Saunders, P. (1993) Citizenship in a liberal society, in *Citizenship and Social Theory*, (ed. B. S. Turner), Sage, London.

Starfield, B. (1994) Is primary care essential? *Lancet*, **344**, 1129–33.

Stern, J. (1983) Social mobility and the interpretation of social class mortality differentials. *Journal of Social Policy*, **12**(1), 27–49.

Stowe, K. (1988) *On Caring For the National Health*, Nuffield Provincial Hospitals Trust, London.

Taylor-Gooby, P. (1985) *Public Opinion, Ideology, and State Welfare*, Routledge and Kegan Paul, London.

Timmins, N. (1996) *The Five Giants*, Fontana, London.

Townsend, P., Davidson, N. and Whitehead, M. (1988) *Inequalities in Health*, Penguin, London.

Wadsworth, M. E. J. (1986) Serious illness in childhood and its association with later life achievement, in *Class and Health: Research and Longitudinal Data*, (ed. R. Wilkinson), Tavistock, London.

Whitehead, M. (1987) *The Growing Health Divide: Inequalities in Health in the 1980s*, Health Education Council, London.

Whitehead, M. (1992) The concepts and principles of equity and health. *International Journal of Health Services*, **2**(3), 429–45.

Whitehead, M. (1994) Who cares about equity in the NHS? *British Medical Journal*, **308**, 1284–7.

Wilkinson, R. (1986) Income and mortality, in *Class and Health: Research and Longitudinal Data*, (ed. R. Wilkinson), Tavistock, London.

Wilkinson, R. (1989) Class and mortality differentials and trends in poverty 1921–1981. *Journal of Social Policy*, **18**, 307–35.

Willetts, D. (1988) Address to the *Financial Times* conference on private health care, London (unpublished).

Willetts, D. and Goldsmith, M. (1988) *Managed Health Care: A New System for a Better Health Service*, Centre for Policy Studies, London.

Key Agencies

Combined trust	Provider unit embracing both hospital(s) and community services
District health authority	Before April 1st 1996, the lower tier health authority (below regional health authority level), responsible for purchasing acute and community health services
GP fundholders	Groups of GPs with budgets for purchasing various categories of health care beyond the primary
Health authority	Since April 1st 1996, the authority responsible for commissioning and purchasing health care (both secondary and primary). Incorporated old district health authorities and family health services authorities (dealing with primary care)
Locality commissioning	Responsibility for purchasing services held below the health authority level, whether led by GPs or others (various forms)
NHS executive	The top management arm of the NHS, within the Department of Health
Regional health authority	Before April 1st 1996, the strategic body responsible for regulating purchasing and provision of health care
Regional office	After April 1st 1996, the division of the NHS executive (a division of the Department of Health) responsible for regulating the purchasing and provision of health care and for carrying out central policies
Trust	Provider with its own board (hospital or other)

Index

Page references in **bold** indicate figures.

Access to services 15–16
Acute trusts
  and community trusts 97, 98
  contracts 79, 80, 82, 85
  and ECRs 96
  information systems 94, **94**, 95, **95**
  see also Hospitals; Providers; Trusts
Adam Smith Institute 23, 25, 26
Allocative efficiency 156
Alma Ata Declaration (1978) 125
Assessment of needs 124–5

Black Report (DHSS 1980) 117, 121
Block contracts 14, 77–8, 78–80, 82–83, 92, 100–1, 102, 153
BMA (British Medical Association) 34, 36, 49
Boards 47–8, 163
Brittan, Leon 24
Bureaucracy
  costs 144–5
  growth 157, 158

Capital
  central priority decisions 32
  charging 31, 32, 41, 147
  future planning 166
  pressure on resources 9
  private 15, 32, 40–1, 41, 174
  public 32, 41, 174
  see also Finance
Catchment areas 11
Centralisation 54
Centre for Policy Studies 25, 26
Charges for services 19, 21
Chief medical officer 29
Clarke, Kenneth 27, 30, 39, 58
  and the BMA 34–5, 36
Collaboration 46, 142–3
Combined trusts
  contracts 79, 80
  and ECRs 96
  information systems 94, **94**, 95, **95**
  see also Providers; Trusts
Commissioning 110–11, 114, 116
  see also Purchasing
Community trusts 15, 30, 66
  and acute trusts 97
  budgets 57
  contracts 79, 80, 82, 84–5
  and ECRs 96
  information systems 94, **94**, 95, **95**
  see also Trusts
Competition 63, 162
  between trusts 9, 98, 143
  managed 17, 32, 133–4
  vs planning 43–4
Consensus management 148
Conservative government (1979–97) 13, 20–1, 114
  see also Prime Minister's Review
Conservative Party 18, 36
Consumer choice 13, 41–2, 141, 159, 163
Contestability 17
Contracts and contracting 9, 10, 31, 63, 72–3
  advantages 105
  causes of failure 92–3, 172
  creation of rigidity in 139
  financially inadequate 152–3
  HA priorities 172

Contracts and contracting (*continued*)
monitoring 91–2, 93
negotiation priorities 87–9
organisation 86–7, **87**, 103
preferred and actual 14, 76–80, **78**, **79**, 80–3, **80**, **81**, 100–1, 102
relationships within 83–6
replacement for 163
and underfunding 55
Cost-per-case contracts 77, 78, 79, 80, 83, 84, 101, 153
Costs 63, 64
bureaucratic 144–5
contracts and 9, 88
labour 8, 9
management 10–11, 12, 13, 56, 147, 156
old and new system comparison 60
of purchaser/provider split 56
of the reforms 99
transactions 60, 135, 136, 144
Cost and volume contracts 77, 82, 83, 84, 100, 153

Diet and health 122
Dobson, Frank 58
Doctors 36
response to White Paper (1989) 34–5
see also GPs
Dorrell, Stephen 49, 58
Drinking and health 122

Economic Affairs, Institute of, Health Unit 21, 22, 25, 26
ECRs *see* Extracontractual referrals
Efficiency 9, 12, 19, 34, 156
'Efficiency trap' 55, 147, 153, 157
Emergency treatment 96–7
Employees *see* Labour
Enthoven, Professor Alain 23, 32–3, 41, 133, 141
Extracontractual referrals (ECRs) 16, 60–2, 95–7, 107, 158

Family Practitioner Committees (FPCs) 49, 50
FHSAs (family health services authorities) 45, 47, 50
Field, Frank 24
Finance
by global cost not contract 166–7
NHS better value than alternative 19
PM's Review and 26–7
possible future 163, 167–8, 170–1
pressure on funding 8
private 15, 18, 32
prospective and retrospective mixture 152–3
public 15, 18, 20, 22
public vs private 168–70
through taxation 7–8
vicious circle of 150
see also Capital
Flexibility, loss of 31
Fundholders *see* GPFHs and fundholding
Funding *see* Finance

General practitioners *see* GPs
Government, central 105
passing the buck 138, 155
setting targets and priorities 12, 116
see also Conservative; Labour
GPFHs (GP fundholders) and fundholding 10, 33–4, 42, 49, 114
allocation of funds 50
benefits and disadvantages 62
contract organisation 86–7, **87**
contract priorities 88–9, **88**, 89
contract relationships 85
contracts and patients 55–6
contract types chosen and preferred 77–8, 78–9, 79–80, **79**, **81**, 83, 100–1
effect on rest of health service 51, 51–2
in the future 51, 62
and HAs 62, 143–4
involvement in planning and purchasing 13, 68, 114–15, 128–30, 166
and market system 137
source of provider income 69, 70, 71
and Trusts 102, 103, 104, 146–7
GPs
1960s–1980s 49–50
budgets 37
changes proposed before PM's Review 23
extending role of 50
giving power to 112
and HAs 144
involvment in purchasing and planning 64, 113, 114–15, 128–30, 165, 166

Labour proposals for 14
and primary care 53
and referrals 31, 61
response to White Paper (1989) 34–5
stress 63
Griffiths Report (1983) 2, 27, 28, 29, 139
Growing Health Divide, The (Whitehead 1987) 117, 123
Guidance in Priorities and Planning for the NHS 1995/96 (NHS Executive) 125
Guy's Hospital 40

Health for All Initiative (WHO 1977) 53
Health Authorities (HAs) 29, 31, 66, 109–10
attitude towards competition 98
boards 47, 48
budgets 41, 67–8, **67**, **68**
catchment areas 11
and contract failures 92–3
contract monitoring 91–2
contract organisation 86, 87, **87**
contract priorities 73–4, 88, **88**, 89, 90
contract relationships 84, 85
contract types chosen 77, **78**, 79, 80, **80**, **81**, 100–1, 102
contract types preferred 81–2, 82, 83, 100–1
co-ordinators of providers 163, 166
and ECRs 96
evolution into purchasers 44–5
and GPFHs 62, 143–4
joint purchasing 91
market structure limitations 68–9
and planning 13
politicisation 35
purchasing function 103–4
source of provider income 69–72
see also Purchasers
Health Care 2000 55, 149
Health insurance 18, 19, 22, 27
Health Maintenance Organisations (HMOs) 133
Health management units (HMUs) 22–3
Health plans 41, 133–4, 141
Health promotion 49, 118, 158
Health status and social class 34, 119–22

Heppel, Strachan 25, 27
Hospitals 30, 52, 66
and community services 15
and contracts 82
funding 158
privatisation 18, 19, 22–3
and trust status 30–1, 32, 33, 40
see also Acute units; Trusts

Inequalities in health 119–24
Infant mortality 120
Information systems 93–5, **94**, **95**, 101
Institute of Economic Affairs, Health Unit 21, 22, 25, 26
Internal market 9, 58, 112
early proposals for 23–4
original intention 32–3
see also Market system

Jenkin, Patrick 20
Joint purchasing 91, 138

Keen, Professor Harry 40

Labour
costs 8, 9
effects of market system 172–3
and 'efficiency' savings 8, 12, 172
morale 63
need for positive incentives 163
planning and training 139
pressures on 9, 63
and private sector 38
Labour government (1997–) 15, 22, 34, 54–5, 117, 135
Labour Party 13–14, 106, 115, 145, 164
Lawson, Nigel 25
Lead providers 43, 44, 97
Local areas/communities
choices instransitive 159
health status 121
involvement in purchasing and planning 115–16, 116–17, 126–8, **127**, 130, 145
and needs assessment 125
Local Freedoms, National Responsibilities (NHS executive 1994) 43, 59
Locality purchasing 105, 129
Local pay 12, 139
Location 99–100
contract priority 73–4

London hospital services 33

McColl, Lord 40
Major, John 25
Management
  complexity 145–6
  costs 10–11, 12, 13, 56, 147, 156
  cuts 173
  investment in and control of 163
  politicisation 35
  reforms 28–30, 148
  separation from planning 45
  use of 12–13
  view of internal market 58–60, 110
Management board, NHS 28
Marketing of services 74–6, **75**
Market system 40, 45–6
  appropriate for NHS 136–7
  conditions for a successful 134–5
  conditions within NHS 135–6
  and the labour force 139
  market as pressure 141
  not a real market in NHS 16–17, 56, 134
  original motivation 141–2
  and planning 11
  politicians and managers views of 9, 58–60
  and productivity 12, 55, 153
  structure limitations 12, 68–9
  see also Internal market
Mawhinney, Dr Brian 43, 109, 126
Moore, John 24, 25, 26, 27
Morale, staff 63
Morbidity rates 120, 121
Mortality rates 120–1, 122

Needs assessment 124–5
Netherlands, The 19, 168, 170
Newton, Tony 25
NHS and Community Care Act (1990) 39, 46
NHS Executive 13, 28, 39, 59, 125
NHS, The: A Service with Ambitions (White Paper) 54
Nichol, Sir Duncan 55, 110, 153

Opinion polls 159
Oregon approach (to rationing) 160
Overprovision 92, 92–3

Paige, Victor 28, 29
Patients
  consumer choice 13, 41–2, 141, 159, 163
  less money for care 156
  money following 31, 54–6
Pay, local 12, 139
Performance indicators 60
Planning 63
  GP involvement 129
  market system and 11, 149
  possible improvements 165–6
  post-reform NHS 113
  pre-reform NHS 111, 112–13
  and purchaser/provider split 43–4
  resurrection of 151
  separating from managment 45
  and strong purchasing 13
  see also Purchasing
Policy board, NHS 28
Politics
  politicisation of NHS 35
  and reforms 2–3, 13
Poverty and health 119, 121, 122–3
Pricing rules 9, 55, 153
Primary care 13, 52–4, 104, 118, 136
Prime Minister's review
  inexperience of reviewers 22
  proposals before 22–5
  stages of 26–8
  structure 25–6
Private finance 15, 32, 140, 174
  vs public 168–70
Private Finance Initiative (PFI) 32, 40–1, 139–40, 148, 174
Private health care 8
  disadvantages 151
  and trusts 38
Private health insurance 7–8, 26, 171
Privatisation 40, 174
  options before 1987 18–19, 21
  proposals before PMs review 22, 22–3
  and purchaser/provider split 148–9
Productivity 12, 55, 63, 153
Profits 171, 172
Promoting Better Health (White Paper 1987) 49
Providers 27–8, 31
  behaviour in the market 134, 135–6
  blamed when things go wrong 107
  competing for contracts 42, 63
  competitive advantages 89–90

contract difficulties 92–3
contract monitoring 91–2, 93
contract negotiations 88–9, **88**
contract organisation 86–7
contract relationships 84–5
contracts at unsustainable rates 172
contract types chosen and preferred 77–80, **78**, **79**, **80**, 81–2, 82–3
co-ordination of 11, 163
determine the services purchased 155–6
and ECRs 96
finance 15, 16, 32, 41, 165
and GPFHs 51, 102, 103, 104, 144
income 68–9, 69–72, **70**
information systems 93–5, **94**, **95**, 101
lead providers 43, 44, 97
local 73–4, 99–100
passing the buck 137, 138, 155
and planning 13, 44, 105, 165
power and influence 14, 57, 58, 72–3, 73
purchasing and 110
and quality 89, 98
relationships between 14–15, 97–8, **97**
relationships with purchasers 12, 99, 101, 143, 144
supplying differing requirements 145–6
see also Purchaser/provider split; Trusts
Public expenditure 8, 9, 149
Public finance 18, 20, 22
vs private 168–70
Public health care
and the better off 150, 168
future prospects 149, 150
views of 8
vs private 170
Public insurance 18, 26, 168–9
Purchaser/provider split 10, 42, 110, 141–2
and buck passing 102
costs and benefits 56–8, 105–6, 107, 144, 157
devolution of 138–9
effects of 86, 104, 153–4, 157
implications for contracting 72–3
and planning 43–4, 45
possible improvements 166
and privatisation 148–9
Purchasers 31, 41, 110
bureaucracy 158
and central government 43, 141
choices constrained 155–6
contract failure causes 92–3
contract organisation 86–7, **87**
contract priorities 73–4, 88–9, **88**, 90
contract relationships 84, 85
contract types chosen 77–80, **78**, **79**, **80**, **81**, 102
contract types preferred 81–2, 82, 83
evolution of HAs into 44–5
finance 15–16, 41
holding back money 157
joint purchasing 91, 138
and local involvement 126–8, **127**
market structure limitations 68–9
objective function 56
passing the buck 137–8, 155
and planning 43–4
power and influence over providers 14, 42, 57, 58, 72
and quality 89, 98
and rationalisation 12, 62
relationships with providers 143
and underfunding 55
see also GPFHs; Health Authorities
Purchasing 109–11, 112, 155
co-ordination 149
decentralising 138–9
GP involvement 128–9
joint 91, 138
local 45, 114, 116, 151
regional 158
separation from service provision 45
strong 13, 109, 110
see also Planning

QALY (Quality of Life Years) 159–60, 160
Quality 92, 98, 105
contract priority 88, 89

Rationalisation 11, 12, 62–3, 106
Rationing 31, 33–4, 55, 153, 159–60
RAWP (resource allocation formula) 21, 32–3, 61
Redwood, John 21, 22
Referrals
extracontractual 16, 60–2, 95–7, 107, 158
and possible future funding 162–3

Referrals (*continued*)
post-reforms 16, 31
pre-reforms 31, 61, 112
Regional offices 2
and planning 13
and rationalisation 12
Regions 24, 32
as purchaser 158
regional funding 31, 165
regional planning 145, 165
resource allocation 111
Resource allocation 41, 115–16, 149, 157
pre-reform NHS 111–12
RAWP formula 21, 32–3, 61
Review, Prime Minister's *see* Prime Minister's Review
Rifkind, Malcolm 25
Right wing ideology 18–19, 24, 40, 141

Secondary care 13, 104, 118, 136
Self-governing hospitals *see* Trusts
Smith, Chris 115
Smoking and health 122
Social class and health 34, 119–22
Social policies, NHS and 117–18, 124, 157–8
Specialised services 104–5, 138
Staff *see* Labour
Stowe, Sir Kenneth 29
Stress 63
Supervisory board, NHS 28
Sweden 19, 121, 170

Taxation 8, 19, 168–9, 171–2
Technical efficiency 156
Thatcher, Margaret 20, 21, 24, 27, 39
see also Prime Minister's review
Towards a Primary-Care Led NHS (NHS Executive) 13
Transactions costs 60, 135, 136, 144
Trusts 12, 66
boards 47, 48, 163
gaining trust status 30–1, 32, 33, 40
and GPFHs 51, 102, 103, 104
politicisation 35
and private purchasers 38
see also Providers

Underfunding 9, 34, 55, 110, 140, 153
USA 133, 170

Voucher systems 22, 159

Waiting lists 31, 62
Waldegrave, William 35, 58
Walker, Peter 25
Whitehead, M. 117, 123
Working conditions and health 123
Working for Patients (White Paper 1989) 1–2, 26, 66
contents 30–2
dangers of 37–8
implementation 32–4
and management of NHS 29–30
politics of 34–5
the real meaning 40–2
working papers 30